# the revival
# slim &
# beautiful
# diet

Say goodbye to belly fat and
hello gorgeous-looking skin, hair, and nails

by Aaron Tabor, MD
and Suzanne Tabor

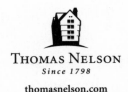

THOMAS NELSON
*Since 1798*

thomasnelson.com

Published in Nashville, Tennessee, by Thomas Nelson, Inc.

Thomas Nelson, Inc. titles may be purchased in bulk for educational, business, fundraising, or sales promotional use. For information, please email SpecialMarkets@ThomasNelson.com.

Published in association with Kevin Small of Result Source, Inc., 7668 El Camino Real, Suite 104716, La Costa, CA 92009.

For marketing partnership inquiries, please contact Physicians Laboratories at Partners@RevivalDiet.com or 1-800-REVIVAL.

Library of Congress Cataloging-in-Publication Data

Tabor, Aaron.
    The revival slim & beautiful diet / by Aaron Tabor and Suzanne Tabor.
        p. cm.
    Includes bibliographical references and index.
    ISBN 10: 0-8499-0355-6 (hardcover)
    ISBN 13: 978-0-8499-0355-7 (hardcover)
    1. Reducing diets. 2. Low-calorie diet. I. Tabor, Suzanne. II. Title. III. Title:
Revival slim and beautiful diet
    RM222.2.R4884 2007
    613.2'5—dc22

                                                        2006101080

Printed in the United States of America
07 08 09 10 11 12 QW 9 8 7 6 5 4 3 2 1

*For my husband, Byran. Any man can be a husband,*
*but it takes a special man to be a best friend.* —*Suzanne*

*For my dad, Byran. Any man can be a father,*
*but it takes a special man to be a dad.* —*Aaron*

# CONTENTS

# ACKNOWLEDGMENTS

Good has greatly blessed us with "First Class" customers, dedicated co-workers, brilliant research colleagues, fabulous friends and a wonderful family. Enjoying good food with you as our good friends makes us clap our hands with joy.

> May the road rise up to meet you.
> May the wind be always at your back.
> May the sun shine warm upon your face;
> the rains fall soft upon your fields
> and until we "meet to eat" again,?
> may God hold you in the palm of His hand.
> —ADAPTED FROM A TRADITIONAL IRISH BLESSING

We've prepared a special video welcome message for you.
Watch it today at **www.RevivalDiet.com**.
Healthy regards,

Suzanne Tabor, "Dr. Mom"

Aaron Tabor, MD

# Please Read for Maximum Results!

We are excited to share with you the wonderful typical results that you can achieve based on numerous Revival clinical trials. The remarkable testimonials we share with you in this book (e.g., a loss of 20 pounds within just a few weeks; dramatic weight drops of 30 to 100 pounds or more; near-total alleviation of PMS or menopausal discomforts; or near-perfect reversal of the visible signs of aging) are not average results, but are included to motivate and inspire you to achieve your dreams!

Average weight loss for the Revival diet study participants was between 26 to 29 ponds in just sixteen weeks. Participants did not experience the typical weight loss "plateau" (i.e., leveling out) seen in many other diets, thus indicating that Revival dieters can continue to lose significant weight well beyond the initial sixteen weeks. Several participants achieved a maximum weight loss of 30 to 40 pounds (or more) during the sixteen-week study, with one participant dropping a stunning 58 pounds.

Remember that, on any diet, nutrition or supplement plan, individual results will vary. Your weight loss results will very based on your starting weight, activity level, and other factors. Revival diet study participants had an average starting weight of about 210 pounds. You need to faithfully follow the restricted-calorie diet plan, regular physical activity plan, and dietary supplement regimens presented in this book if you hope to achieve great weight loss, beauty, and health results documented in numerous Revival studies and other clinical trials. Typical results you can expect are discussed for each Revival study.

Your well-being is extremely important to us. Because this diet is so powerful at producing rapid weight loss, do not try to lose more than 2 pounds per week or eat less than 1200 calories per day, unless you are under the supervision of your healthcare provider. A healthy weight loss rate is typically 1 to 2 pounds per week. Rapid weight loss may lead to health problems.

For maximum results, discuss this diet and information with your healthcare provider, especially if you are trying to lose more than 30 pounds, have special medical dietary needs, suffer with a chronic medical condition, take prescription medication, are under eighteen, pregnant, or nursing.

Of course, Revival's research information and products do not take the place of your healthcare provider's advice, nor do they substitute for prescription medication, surgery, chemotherapy, radiation therapy, or any other medical treatment. These statements have not been evaluated by the Food and Drug Administration. Revival is not intended to diagnose, treat, cure, or prevent any disease.

In other words, use some common sense when it comes to your health! *Let's get started!*

**FACT:** The power and simplicity of *The Revival Slim & Beautiful Diet* rescued my mom, and it can also help you. It is a clinically proven "nutritional makeover" to help dieters lose 26 to 29 pounds on average in just sixteen weeks and to dramatically improve skin, hair, and nail appearance.

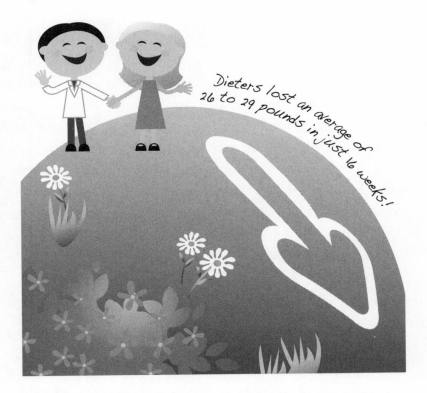

Dieters lost an average of 26 to 29 pounds in just 16 weeks!

Together we will fight an all-out nutritional war against ugly, "gelatinous" fat (particularly belly fat!), low energy, appearance of wrinkles, dull hair, and weak nails.

Hi, I'm Dr. Tabor. If you are fed up with how you look and feel, then let's take a simple walk down the hill together to a "slim and beautiful" new you!

## CHAPTER 1

# A Doctor-Designed Diet that Rescued Mom™

M ay I have a dessert menu?"

These are the shocking words I recently overheard an overweight woman ask her waitress. Why was I shocked? Because she had just devoured a gigantic plate of pancakes saturated with strawberry syrup and topped with a tall spire of whipped cream as her "dinner." Did I mention the quarter-pound of sausage she also inhaled? Houston, we have a problem . . . a really "big" problem.

It honestly broke my heart for her.

As a medical research doctor and graduate from The Johns Hopkins School of Medicine, I've dedicated my life to discovering *easy* ways for people to lose weight, look beautiful, and live healthy, empowered lives.

It is painful for me to see someone making food their master, serving it *versus* letting food serve them with beautifying nutrition, as it was designed to do! I believe every day is a gift, and our eating should reflect our gratefulness for life.

If your weight and appearance are preventing you from living a life you absolutely love. I am here to help you. This clinically proven diet is designed to produce slim and beautiful bodies, but if you are only trying to look better in a bathing suit, we have some deep priority issues to resolve. Why? Because

I know your excess fat is killing you—and that's a little more important than how you look in a bathing suit.

---

**FACT:** Being fat doesn't *bite* the hand
that feeds you—it *kills* it!

---

So, if you are looking for undying sympathy because overeating has made you gelatinous, it won't come from me. However, if you need a friend to empower you with clinically proven truth and advice, then I am here with my hand raised high! I will be with you every step of the way down a new "nutritional makeover" path.

Like our moms said, "Sometimes the truth hurts," but our acknowledging the truth is the only way we can walk and work together hand-in-hand towards *drastically* changing how you look and feel.

---

**FACT:** You are fat because you choose to be.

---

I'm not going to sugar-coat the facts-about-fat for you: You are fat because you have *chosen* to be fat by eating more calories than you burn.

Sadly, your chosen path leads to more than thirty deadly diseases, such as breast cancer, ovarian cancer, high blood pressure, high cholesterol, diabetes, stroke, and sudden-death heart attack. A fat life *is* like a box of chocolates: you never know what disease you are going to get.

Death walks slowly toward all of us from birth, but when we are fat, death *runs* toward us. We don't even have to move off our couches! The big bad wolf will break your little piggy door down sooner or later—it's a fact.

Have you already failed on another diet? It's okay; I have too. More than likely, the diet failed you instead of you failing the diet. What I mean is that many popular diets have never actually been clinically proven to work in a well-designed clinical trial. You end up feeling hungry, constantly hungry, which leads to another dismal diet failure.

Unfortunately, many popular diets are also too difficult to be understood easily unless you have a science degree. Complicated or controversial theories produce more confusion than lost pounds. Even worse than a confusing diet plan is a plan that is too complex to continue using over time, making the minimal results you achieve short-lived. After suffering on the diet for a few weeks, you "fall off the wagon," and the pounds rush back to your belly, *gluteus maximus*, and legs, clinging on in clumps of dietary defiance. Having the "max" return to your *maximus* isn't fun or flattering.

Sound familiar? Well, I've eliminated these traditional diet problems with a super simple, yet extremely powerful, diet and physical activity plan. Take a big breath and relax because it is proven to work. We will jump full speed into the plan in the next chapter.

## DO YOU HAVE A DREAM OF A BEAUTIFUL, HEALTHY LIFE YOU ACTUALLY LOVE?

Developing a clear vision of your dream body and life is important for you to succeed. If all you have are visions of sugarplums dancing in your head, you will continue to be "plump." The hero Dr. Jonas Salk, inventor of the polio vaccine, made a profound statement, "I have had dreams and I have had nightmares, but I have conquered my nightmares because of my dreams."

You and I can conquer your beauty and weight nightmares and make your dreams a reality because of new medical research.

**FACT:** Your past diet failures no longer determine your future, because new beauty research developments exist.

You are going to learn about specific solutions that I've created and helped research in this book. I believe you will find it infinitely more helpful than the general diet and nutrition information found in hundreds of other diet books. I've spent seven years developing *The Revival Slim & Beautiful Diet* at some of America's best hospitals. The diet is based on numerous Revival medical studies, including National Institutes of Health (NIH) funded work on Revival's role in promoting normal cholesterol levels. Revival is doctor-approved— *thousands* of physicians have already recommended Revival products, and several hundred thousand people have become customers (affectionately called "Revival-LITES" by mom and me). Many brilliant medical researchers, whom I am honored to call my colleagues, have contributed to this research (in particular Dr. James Anderson and Dr, Robert Blair). Our medical research continues to make more discoveries for you. We are working diligently to bring many good things to your life.

## "ASK NOT WHAT YOUR BODY CAN DO FOR YOU; ASK WHAT YOU CAN DO FOR YOUR BODY."

If we treat our bodies well, they will take us to some amazing places in life. Our bodies are the ultimate driving machines.

Let's see a vision of where we are headed to, as we walk down the hill together.

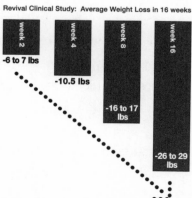

Revival Clinical Study: Average Weight Loss in 16 weeks

week 2 — -6 to 7 lbs

week 4 — -10.5 lbs

week 8 — -16 to 17 lbs

week 16 — -26 to 29 lbs

Dieters in Revival's weight loss clinical trial, conducted at a major independent academic hospital, achieved spectacular average results by enjoying Revival's milk-protein-based diet or soy-protein-based diet.[†] The diet plan combined with the activity plan detailed in this book is designed to help dieters:

- lose 26 to 29 pounds in just sixteen weeks (about 1 to 2 pounds per week);
- quickly reduce gelatinous belly fat (lose up to 25 percent or more in sixteen weeks), shrink your waist circumference, and lose dress/pant sizes;
- reduce hunger and satisfy sweet, salty, and crunchy cravings;
- promote better energy levels with protein-packed, low-glycemic "smart-carb" choices (i.e., no rapid rise in blood sugar levels);
- promote normal cholesterol levels;
- promote normal blood pressure;
- maintain proper blood sugar levels.

With Revival's soy-protein-based diet (that includes special naturally concentrated Revival products discussed in the next chapter), medical research shows additional health and "nutritional makeover" beauty benefits.[†] Individual results vary, but the plan is designed to:

- reduce appearance of wrinkles with less roughness and better coloration;
- increase hair silkiness with reduced dullness and better manageability;
- strengthen nails with less splitting, ridging, and flaking;

---

[†]Individual results vary. You must follow the calorie-restricted diet plan, physical activity plan, and dietary supplement regimens in this book if you hope to achieve great weight loss, beauty, and health results. See the *Introduction* and specific studies presented in this book for typical results. These statements have not been evaluated by the Food and Drug Administration. Revival is not intended to diagnose, treat, cure, or prevent any disease.

- balance hormones for reduced hot flashes, night sweats, and lessened PMS;
- maintain healthier tissues with natural soy antioxidants;
- support normal memory and cognition health;
- promote better bone health.

Do these diet benefits sound too good to be true? Could a simple plan really produce powerful results? Well, it's time to tell your inner Mr. Doubt to simply "tear down these walls," and let medical research truth set you free.

Why would I work for seven years researching and perfecting this diet? Because of a special woman—Suzanne Tabor—my wonderful mom! I'm privileged to co-write this book with her because she is an amazing mother, wife (she and dad recently celebrated forty-one years together), and businesswoman. If there were a Nobel Prize for parenting, my parents definitely deserve it for successfully raising three boys. "Dr. Mom" has that wholesome Southern down–to–earth goodness that immediately puts you at ease. I'm happy that you get to "meet" her shortly. She will share her "Bright Bites" with us throughout the book to inspire us and make us laugh. She has already walked down the hill to a better place. And, if I know my mom, she is making us a healthy picnic lunch to enjoy upon arrival.

At fifty years old, my mom was a wreck in the midst of a midlife meltdown. A rapidly enlarging waistline embarrassed her. Clothes that used to fit were now uncomfortable. Unrelenting hot flashes and night sweats (sometimes fifty per day) disrupted her work, concentration, and sleep. Low energy hovered like a dark cloud over her day, making routine tasks seem impossible. Deepening wrinkle appearance, dull hair, weak nails, and dry skin were not only a very uncomfortable annoyance, but were also taking a deep emotional toll on her self-esteem.

To make things worse, hormone-related moods swings began disrupting her otherwise harmonious marriage with my dad. We all know it's true that if mom isn't happy, no one is happy. At one point, Dad started singing, "Don't Be Cruel" and "You've Lost that Loving Feeling" in his off-key voice.

He unfortunately didn't improve the situation when he blurted out in frustration, "You need anti-Tasmanian Devil medication!" Ouch! He obviously had not paid attention to mom's favorite coffee cup: "I'm out of estrogen and I have a gun!"

When mom called me insisting for help, I knew from the sound of her tearfully stressed-out voice that something very special and very powerful had to be done to help her. Most great moms are very picky, and mine is no exception. Not only did she want a solution, it needed to be a natural solution for her worsening situation.

If you are blessed with great parents who make you proud, then you know precisely how painful it is to see them suffer with anything, big or small. To see my mom—the mom I always give a "World's Best Mom" card to on Mother's Day—totally beaten down physically and emotionally was alarming.

Her midlife "tribulations" fueled my unrelenting quest to develop a natural solution to rescue her. After all, it was *my* mom enduring this burden! Something had to be done to fix it. Multiple years of research has led me to create Revival products (both milk-protein-based and soy-protein-based products) and to develop *The Revival Slim & Beautiful Diet*—a delicious, doctor-designed solution engineered for total body beauty and wellness. (And, yes, the diet includes chocolate in case you are wondering!) They say necessity is the mother of invention. I say, "My mother necessitated the invention."

Mom is doing fabulously now with tons of energy (she has more than I do!), a slim and svelte waistline, balanced hormones, free of the Tasmanian Devil, and beautiful-looking skin, hair, and nails. Everyone comments on how her skin glows with a smooth radiant appearance (which needless to say makes her feel great about herself), and how healthy and silky her long hair is. To be honest, I think she is more excited about her stronger nails and softer skin than her smaller dress size and minimized hot flashes and night sweats. And for me, a medical research doctor, it is rewarding to know that the diet supports her normal heart and bone health. That makes me happy.

As for my dad, he is once again on cloud nine, an incredibly blessed man. After escaping mom's dog house by profusely apologizing for his unwise medication comments, he is singing "My Girl" to his tempting bride.

He and I both follow the diet daily, too, in case you are wondering. And neither of us have had a single hot flash in seven years! But all joking aside, all is well in Tabor-ville.

Mom says, "Revival gave me my life back!"

My dad chimes in, "Revival gave me my *wife* back!"

We've all suffered through bad events, including sickness, lost of a loved one, or a broken heart. It's an unavoidable part of life. Sometimes the purpose of our suffering isn't clear. But in this case, Mom and I both understand exactly why she had to endure such health and beauty tribulations: Because of mom's *temporary* situation, she and I have now been blessed to help thousands of people live a life they love with Revival. It's a very humbling role that we consider an honor to fulfill. Waking up every day knowing that we are actively helping tens of thousands of people (and more every day) is a top-of-the-world feeling.

Mom and I want to help you create a life and body that you love, too.

---

**FACT:** Beauty is only skin deep,
but unhealthiness goes all the way to your bones.

---

This "Mom-approved" diet plan covertly helps you do something even more important than improving your outward appearance—it helps support your entire body's health from the inside out.

What good is a slim waistline or beautiful skin, hair, and nails if your heart is too frail for you to walk, or your bones so unhealthy that you stoop over with your face to the ground?

This diet is designed to do so much more for you than to simply make you pretty. I often call *The Revival Slim & Beautiful Diet* the "diet *plus* plan" because it helps you lose weight and look great, *plus* it may help balance your hormones to reduce common discomforts of PMS and menopause; *plus* it may help promote healthy bones; *plus* it may support normal memory and cognition health; *plus* it may promote energy with protein-packed, low-glycemic benefits; *plus* it may promote maintenance of proper blood sugar levels; *plus* it bathes your body and skin in antioxidants; and, *plus* it may promote normal blood pressure health and normal cholesterol levels (which may reduce your risk of heart disease, the number-one killer of women and men). You are in good hands with the Revival Slim and Beautiful Diet.

You do not need a math degree to understand that these health benefits add up for your happiness, but you do need to understand that a critical decision must be made today, a decision which is the most important part of this diet equation:

*Are you ready to take the first steps in creating your beautiful dream body and life you love?*

If you can't say an emphatic "yes!" today, I believe you are destined for a short-lived future, troubled by accelerated health problems and continued deterioration of your beauty.

I promise that if you choose to start walking down a new path with me today, you will enjoy a slim and beautiful new you—healthier and sexier than ever. So, if you are tired of looking fat with a dull appearance and feeling even worse, I'm asking you to start down the hill with me—today.

Do you believe every day is a gift, as I do? If you do, take the first step *today*—it's important because that means we've already won half of the nutritional war against ugly fat and wrinkles. I believe you want to make the right decision because you know how unhealthy, and even deadly, being fat can be.

Today's decision is not only one small step for your weight, but one giant leap toward a beautiful life you will love.

Put on your "diet boots" made for walking.

*Let's meet mom and then get a move on!*

## MEET MY MOM!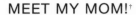

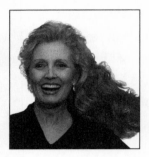

Greetings!

I'm Suzanne, Aaron's mom. I call him "Doc." He says he likes to call me "Dr. Mom" because I've helped him so much during his life. If you have raised a child (I've raised three), you understand that we moms deserve an honorary medical degree!

I decided to help him write this book because I truly hope it will be good news to you, and will lighten your load (literally and mentally).

Doc's a no-nonsense, don't-give-me-any-measly-excuses type of person, so I'm here to cushion the journey. And I hope to make the trip more fun, as all good moms do. Above all, I want my personal health success story to be an inspiring encouragement to you.

Let me assure you that there is hope for you, whatever the situation.

Are you tired, discouraged, or just plain worn out? Take heart, I understand what it's like to feel that way, whether you are young or old. At age fifty I was a wreck!

Fifty is a fine number, unless it represents the number of hot flashes you're having each night, or the number of steps it takes you to wear out, or the dress size you fear may be yours. This is not much of an exaggeration for the condition I felt my life was in.

I thought after I raised the kids I would be kicking up my heels with my handsome hunk of a husband, but I was too busy fanning my face during the day and desperately tossing off the sheets at night.

When I called Doc to tell him of the hormonal tornado sweeping through my body and our once-peaceful home, I was at the end of my rope men-

---

tally and physically. I know my husband probably felt like he was hanging from the same rope because of my roller-coaster mood swings. My shrinking physical health, combined with my expanding waistline, started taking a toll on my emotions. My self-esteem became "less pretty" as my skin, hair, and nails started looking worn. My mom had always told me there would be bad days, but she didn't tell me they could be this bad!

I definitely wasn't anywhere close to living a life I love. In fact, I was so far away that I couldn't even see a light at the end of the tunnel. My "balanced diet" had become a chocolate chip cookie in each hand. I soon found out that eating what I wanted and praying to not gain weight didn't work.

Midlife had finally knocked me on my fat behind and back. I felt trapped in a worsening "Hormonal Hades."

I reached out to my son for help; actually, I *insisted* that he help. I felt like the flood victims we see on television, the ones on top of the rooftop with the water raging around their shambled home while they grasp to survive until the helicopter arrives. I knew my firm foundation was nearly eroded, and my "home" would collapse soon. My husband got on the phone with Doc to express his concern that something had to be done quickly.

Call it woman's intuition, but a natural solution felt like just the thing my mind and body needed, so that is what I asked Doc to create. Thank God for using my son to create Revival. For years, I was thinking, "By the time I'm thin, fat will be in."

*Revival gave me my hope back and my health back.* It restored my foundation firmly. I suddenly had more energy without feeling hungry, and my menopausal discomforts nearly vanished in four weeks. I now have the best skin, hair, and nail appearance of my life and a slim waistline that I love.

*I'm confident and in control again.* So maybe I don't feel eighteen years old again, but I feel pretty close to forty—which is plenty enough improvement for me. Over time, I feel as though Revival has turned back the clock on my parched body.

Who would have dreamed when I entered midlife that my health burdens and Doc's persistence would end up producing not only a solution for my woes, but also a company that helps thousands to feel better every day? My prayer of desperation was answered in ways I could never have dreamed of—indeed, God gave new purpose to my midlife experience. Nothing was wasted.

What is your hope today? To feel better? To have more energy? To slim down? To look vibrant and young? To have normal cholesterol levels? To stop feeling like a walking human heat lamp? To stop feeling so grouchy? To feel joyful more often? To love more, help others, and find significant purpose?

It happened for me, and it can happen for you, too, one small step, one small change, and one small page of this book at a time. Why am I certain? Because the diet is delicious (and Doc gets an A+ from me for including so much chocolate). For me to use any diet or product, for ten seconds or ten years, it has to be full of great flavor. I've been using Revival for ten years now. And I believe that life's too short to ever eat bad-tasting food. Revival truly did give me my life back. I love my new and improved look.

Call it a mother's heart, but I wish I could talk with each of you personally to offer my encouragement and a hug. If you want to share your own stories and thoughts with me, e-mail me at **Mom@RevivalDiet.com**.

*Never ever give up on your hopes and dreams.* Don't forget that dieting is "wishful shrinking." My son's research made it easy for me, and you can have what you wish for, too.

I'll be here to cheer you up and cheer you on because I understand where you currently are in life. But more importantly, I understand where you can and should be. Some laughter mixed with words of wisdom from Mom is still the best medicine.

Walk the good walk while you press on!

## CHAPTER 2

# Rapid Weight Loss Plan: *The Revival Slim & Beautiful Diet*

*Every beauty which is seen here below by persons of perception resemble more than anything else that celestial source from which we all are come.*
—MICHELANGELO (1475–1564)

So, here we are with our diet boots on, ready to start down the hill.

> **FACT:** Successful dieting is not about constantly denying or punishing yourself.

Successful dieting *is* about finding delicious foods that 1) you absolutely love, and 2) empower you to lose weight.

Based on my years of medical research, I believe that you are going to love this clinically proven plan. But don't just take my word for it. Before we start, how does a pre-walk "pep talk" from real, unpaid Revival-LITES sound?

*My skin looks more radiant than ever. Does Revival get all of the credit? I think so! Besides, I'm not willing to stop Revival to find out differently!*

—H. B. HOFFMANN, Results not typical.[†]

*Revival has transformed my life! My days were plagued by hot flashes, broken nails, and limp hair, plus I was overweight. Now I am 24 pounds lighter, my hair and nails are not brittle, and my hot flashes are less frequent. I feel like a new woman, young and vital. I do not look fifty-two years old. Thank you Revival. I am most grateful for this new lease on life.*

—Z. ROSENBAUM, Results not typical.[†]

*My dermatologist comments on the toned look and dewiness of my skin since I have been on Revival. She's actually recommending it to her patients. My hair is shinier and in better condition also. I have more energy and feel stronger.*

—C. KUSHKIN, Results not typical.[†]

*Wow!! . . . I have been steadily losing weight since the beginning of the year. I have gone down three to four dress/pant sizes! My weight loss has been about 35 pounds. At forty-one years old, I have never felt better. (And I look much better than most of my friends. I am the envy of my high school graduation gang.) I had a life-long weight problem and now I have gone from a size 14 to a size 4 or 6 in about eight months. Looking for a spokesmodel?*

—K. DEBUSK, NP, Results not typical.[†]

Ready to start walking down the hill together to join the others? Let's "stretch our legs" and dreams with a few more encouraging testimonies before we start:

---

[†]Results not typical, but included to motivate you. Individual results vary. You must follow the calorie-restricted diet plan, physical activity plan, and dietary supplement regimens presented in this book if you hope to achieve great weight loss, beauty, and health results. see *Introduction* and specific studies presented in this book for typical results. These statements have not been evaluated by the Food and Drug Administration. Revival is not intended to diagnose, treat, cure, or prevent any disease.

*I didn't know Revival would improve my skin and hair, so it was quite a nice surprise after about three months to see such a difference. Friends say I never looked better.*

—T. TEED, Results not typical.[†]

*Eating Revival, along with a walking program, I have been able to shed these 60 pounds with no uncontrollable cravings for food.*

—S. J. HOLCOMBE, Results not typical.[†]

*My OB/GYN doctor thought I should try Revival. She has been using it herself for some time. Well, I love it! My skin feels smoother. I have more energy. Revival fills me up, and I do not want sweets. Thank you.*

—S. BASTIANELLI, Results not typical.[†]

We've all seen her. She's worked hard, lost weight, and is expectantly waiting for us to tell her how beautiful she looks. But her skin has lost its glow, her fine lines replaced with deepening appearance of wrinkles, and in places her discolored skin even sags. Her hair shows the telltale signs of dullness. Her nails are weak and brittle and her eyes tired. She looks so weak you want to offer her a place to put her feet up and rest along with a good wholesome meal. It's the look of someone who's lost weight at a concentration camp, and though you may admire her fortitude, her will power, and her endurance, you must admit, at least to yourself, "This is not pretty."

Forrest Gump's mother, along with my own Southern mom, had a saying, "Pretty is as pretty does." Turns out that this not only means that beauty comes from a well-watered soul and kind spirit, it also comes from what we put into our bodies—much more than the lotions we slather on them. Physical beauty is more than skin deep; it starts with nourishing our bodies through what we eat and drink. Simply put, the higher our intake of the world's most nutritious foods, the more our bodies will become lean, beautiful, energized, and healthy. And that's a fact, based on the best research available today. I'll show you exactly how to lose weight while improving your appearance, instead of destroying your appearance.

Staying slim and beautiful during our twenties and thirties is already difficult enough today, given the abundance of tantalizing temptations and cream puff pitfalls. Even worse, the approach to midlife brings about additional challenges—pressures to keep a youthful appearance, aging parents, an empty nest, retirement planning, and more. This new stress coupled with reduced physical activity and fluctuating hormones can exacerbate weight gain and cause drastic negative changes in skin, hair, and nail appearance. So, if you've noticed that the needle on your scale keeps creeping to the right and your appearance is losing its luster, you're not alone. Yes, those are pounds showing on your scale, not ounces!

## MOM'S BRIGHT BITE

You know it is time to diet and exercise during midlife when your children look through your wedding album and want to know who Dad's first wife was! It wasn't quite that bad for me, but you get the picture. Our bodies change dramatically as we age, so we can't take our great shape from earlier years for granted. If you wait too long to start taking better care of yourself, you will find that your fat has become best friends with your body!

Let me explain my passion a bit. As a graduate of a research-oriented medical school—it was a real blessing and dream to be educated at Johns Hopkins—I am not a big fan of touchy-feely approaches to life. I am, and have always been, a "just give me the facts, ma'am" kind of guy. I love discovering the truth through medical research and then using that truth to makes someone's life more beautiful. I am blessed to have loving parents who taught me the value of hard, persistent work coupled with the importance of finding truth in a world troubled by illusions. If I have an addiction, I must admit, it would be working to find the world's most efficient and healthiest fuels to beautify and run these amazing bodies God created—and to save the world from eating itself into an ugly, early grave. I'm sort of a Dr. Phil-meets-Hippocrates man, with a touch of super-hero save-and-beautify-the-planet passion burning in my mind and soul.

I *am* here to "save the day," or I should say to save your days.

Most people hate it when I choose to use the word "gelatinous" instead of the word "fat." I choose gelatinous because it isn't a pretty image. Defined by Webster's Medical Dictionary as "resembling gelatin or jelly," I hope it invokes a more repulsive picture in your mind than simply "fat" or "overweight." The Pillsbury Doughboy is "fat," but he's round, smooth, and cute. When we humans are overweight, our belly and body fat isn't round, smooth, or cute—it's "gelatinous"—and deadly! I don't know about you, but the thought of billions of fat cells clumping together in my body makes me lose my appetite. Cuddly little fat cells are about as cute as little deadly bacteria and viruses. Get the picture? Let it motivate you to remodel yourself.

## MOM'S BRIGHT BITE

Being able to laugh at yourself is a healthy step in the right direction because it means you have more control over yourself.

I found my gelatinous body (I hate that word, too) did offer some advantages—since I can't swim that well! All joking aside, your "life preserver" should be a healthy heart, brain, and bones, not fat that floats.

As a result of seeing Revival give my mom the best health and beauty of her life, I founded Physicians Laboratories where I am CEO and Medical Research Director. Our company's mission is to serve others with good nutrition, education, and medical research so they can live a life they love. Mom and I work side-by-side on a daily basis; she is my president and chief financial officer (CFO) with the self-proclaimed additional job duty of finding me a great wife (which she frequently mentions to office visitors!)

---

## MOM'S BRIGHT BITE

A husband of a Revival customer called us to say, "I don't know what you are sending my wife, but don't stop! She's acting like she's eighteen again!"

---

With nearly thirty clinical trials underway or completed, we are accomplishing our company's mission by producing the best clinically proven products that make weight loss and beauty *super easy* for the average person. (I'll tell you about the products and what a typical day will look like for you on this diet in just a moment.) As part of my research work, I've been blessed to make health discoveries that are now patented in eleven different countries (and growing) including the United States, England, Italy, France, and even China.

As I studied a solution for my mom's midlife meltdown, including her weight gain and deepening wrinkle appearance, I was amazed at the complicated diet plans being pushed in the marketplace. Most popular diet plans are difficult to learn, hard to use, and impossible to stay on long-term. I was more amazed, and even disturbed, to learn that most popular diets were created by good marketing, not good science. Also, I could not find a diet that was actually *clinically proven* to improve the appearance of skin, hair, and nails in a clinical trial. When I investigated other diet "prescriptions" for better skin, I found they were only speculations with little-to-no supporting evidence. I found myself asking, "Where's the proof?"

Sick and tired of marketing illusions, I decided to do something about it by creating *The Revival Slim & Beautiful Diet*, a clinically proven plan that's easy to learn, simple to use, and enjoyable to stay on long-term. It's realistic.

If you are like 90 percent of people I know (including my mom), you are too busy to tediously count calories day after day after day, manage complex phase ins and phase outs, or constantly shop to prepare gourmet recipes with the "right" balance of carbohydrates. You also realize that unrealistic dietary demands, such as eliminating all carbs or eating fat-free, are not only impossible, but detrimental to your overall health and success. You don't believe that bread and pasta are evil, and neither do I.

All that you want is a simple, pleasurable diet plan to help you lose weight, feel energized and look beautiful—without feeling constantly hungry and without having all of your food choices and family eating time stripped away from you.

You also don't want to risk your health by using dangerous diet pills hawked all over late night television, touting unproven, often ridiculous claims. Who hasn't heard about the "Lose 10 pounds in one weekend" juice diet?

## MOM'S BRIGHT BITE

Laughter is great diet medicine. Did you hear about the new creative way doctors are forcing patients to get more exercise? "I'm prescribing these pills for you," said the doctor to the overweight patient who refused to exercise. "I don't want you to swallow them. Just spill them on the floor twice a day and pick them up, one at a time."

This just proves that relying on pills to lose weight is not a smart idea!

Sure, a woman may starve herself to lose ten pounds of water weight to fit into that clingy red dress for a glitzy party. But we know she'll put those pounds back on, once the dress is off, faster than you can say "Twinkies." I heard a comedian say that fast-food companies are considering including special toys with their supersized heart-attacks-in-sacks: little miniature tombstones! Many a truth is spoken in jest, or as William Shakespeare wrote in *King Lear* more than four hundred years ago, "Jesters do oft prove prophets."

You, like the rest of us, are sick and tired of looking and feeling sick and tired.

This is your diet plan because you can have it your way and love it with delicious foods that satisfy your hunger and heal your appearance.

---

### MOM'S BRIGHT BITE

The problem with curbing our appetites is that most of us do it at the drive-in window of our favorite fast food restaurants!

---

## "I'M READY TO START LOSING. FEED ME THE DETAILS!"

You *can* enjoy immediate results including the loss of ugly belly fat on the *Revival Slim and Beautiful Diet*. It is clinically proven to help dieters lose an average 6 to 7 pounds in just two weeks. That's almost one clingy, little red dress size! And the results don't have to stop there.

Let me share a motivational chart with you showing what's possible based on the results of Revival's clinical trial at a major independent academic hospital using Revival's simple milk-protein-based diet or soy-protein-based diet, combined with the physical activity plan detailed in this chapter. Several dieters achieved a maximum weight loss of 30 to 40 pounds (or more) during the sixteen-week study, while the average dieter still enjoyed these incredible results:

## AVERAGE WEIGHT LOSS RESULTS

- Lost **3** to **4** pounds in one week (several participants lost more than **5** pounds).
- Lost **6** to **7** pounds in two weeks (several participants lost more than **8** pounds).
- Lost **10.5** pounds in four weeks (several participants lost more than **12** pounds).
- Lost **14** pounds in six weeks (several participants lost more than **17** pounds).
- Lost **16** to **17** pounds in eight weeks (several participants lost more than **20** pounds).
- Lost **26** to **29** pounds in sixteen weeks (several participants lost more than **40** pounds).
- Lost **25** percent of belly fat in sixteen weeks.
- Reduced waist circumference by 12 percent in sixteen weeks.

Just so you know, these are amazing weight loss results, but not "ridiculous" results because the plan is based on sound medical research. To put these results into perspective, they are among the very best ever published in a peer-reviewed medical journal.

Because this diet is so powerful at producing rapid weight loss, I recommend that you do not try to lose more than 2 pounds per week or consume less than 1200 calories per day, unless you are under the supervision of your healthcare provider.

You wouldn't want to take off in a powerful rocket without an expert co-pilot, so if you are trying to lose a large amount of weight quickly, make sure your healthcare provider is on board with you. Your healthcare provider will likely recommend that you aim for 1 to 2 pounds of weight loss per week with at least 1200 calories per day.

Why limit your "rocket speed"? Because losing more than 2 pounds per week or eating less than 1200 calories per day for an extended period of time can increase your risk of exhaustion, dehydration, or nutrient deficiencies, leading to illness or injury. Burning too much fuel too soon isn't wise if we want to successfully complete the mission.

The dieters in the sixteen-week clinical trial started out with an average weight of about 210 pounds, so they obviously had a large amount of fat to lose (for the intellectually curious, participants' average Body Mass Index [BMI] was 35.) You don't have to be a rocket scientist to know that your weight loss results will vary based on your starting weight and your long-term faithfulness to the diet and physical activity plan. Achieve amazing results by being faithful.

If you do want to lose more than 2 pounds per week, you and your healthcare provider can easily modify the diet plan to lower your calorie intake to less than 1200 calories per day. I'll show you how later in the chapter.

Remember that we want to *walk* down the hill, not *roll* down the hill! Rolling down a hill is not a pretty sight.

## THE WEIGHT JUST KEEPS GOING, AND GOING, AND GOING . . .

The good news is that the Revival diet study data suggests you can lose as many pounds as you want to lose, whether 20 pounds or 200 pounds, *over time* by persistently using this plan. In other words, if you are faithful to the diet and physical activity plan you can keep losing weight every week well beyond sixteen weeks until you arrive beautifully at your dream destination.

**FACT:** Revival dieters in the clinical trial did not show the signs of every dieter's nightmare— the dreaded plateau that typically happens within a few weeks after starting a new diet.

During a plateau, weight loss inexplicably levels out. It just suddenly stops and additional weight loss is very difficult. Remarkably, the Revival dieters continued to lose weight at virtually the same rapid pace (nearly 2 pounds per week) during the entire study from Week 1 all the way through Week 16.

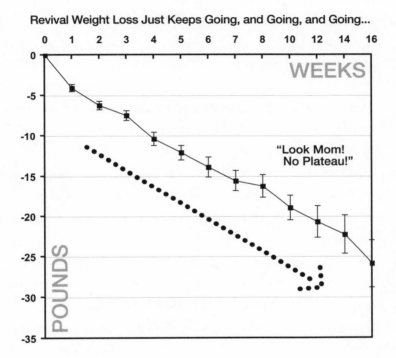

**Revival Weight Loss Just Keeps Going, and Going, and Going...**

Are you ready to conquer your diet nightmares for the sake of your beautiful dreams? You can when you are empowered with the right medical research. Most of us have experienced hitting this proverbial weight loss wall. The pounds are falling off until suddenly our weight-loss rocket stalls and falls, with no more results no matter what we try. Some of us have even shaken our weight loss scales in disbelief and frustration to make sure they aren't broken!

Well, this diet is designed to be so super simple to understand, use, and enjoy, so that your weight loss just keeps going, and going, and going! You find your hunger reduced and your willpower *energized* (just like the bunny—will someone please stop him from beating that drum?).

---

### MOM'S BRIGHT BITE

You know it is time to be serious about eating healthy to shed the pounds when you step on a talking scale and it says, "Only one person is allowed on the scale at a time!

---

## WHAT EXPLAINS THE CONTINUED RAPID WEIGHT LOSS?

The explanation is easy—the Revival dieters *used* the diet consistently during the entire study, even all the way through the last week. *The Revival Slim & Beautiful Diet* is easy, delicious and *satisfying*—which is a definite recipe for long-term diet success.

This is the right diet using the right products; that's why I'm so passionate about it. A diet is worthless if it isn't simple and delicious enough to be used and enjoyed over an extended amount of time. People simply refuse to stay on a complicated diet using products they don't love. The pounds pop off and then pop back on. Has yo-yo dieting jerked you around and beaten you down in the past?

Don't worry. I have your back covered . . . and your belly, thighs, and *gluteus maximus* with the *Revival Slim and Beautiful Diet*. Let's see how to turn your *maximus* into *minimus* right now!

## RAPID WEIGHT LOSS USING THE REVIVAL SLIM AND BEAUTIFUL DIET

*Simplicity is the ultimate sophistication.*
—LEONARDO DA VINCI

Simplicity is the true beauty of this diet. There are no complicated theories to memorize, or crazy tactics to leave you hungry and tired.

The moment has finally arrived to share the plan with you . . . the simple, proven directions for walking the downhill path to a slim and beautiful new you . . . *drumroll please!*

---

## HOW TO ACHIEVE RAPID WEIGHT LOSS

Here's how a rapid weight loss day would look:

1. Enjoy 2 to 3 Revival milk-protein or soy-protein bars and shakes.
2. Enjoy 5 servings of fruits and vegetables of your choice.
3. Enjoy 1 low-calorie meal or pre-packaged entrée of your choice.

**BONUS SNACKS:** Enjoy 2 Revival snacks substituted for 1 bar or shake.

That's it for the eating plan.

---

We will discuss details about the bars, shakes, entrées, fruits and vegetables, and snacks shortly, but if at any time you need help understanding the diet, products, or planning your daily eating pattern below, please don't hesitate to contact my friendly nutrition staff at **1-800-REVIVAL** (1-800-738-4825), **www.RevivalDiet.com,** or Nutrition@RevivalDiet.com.

## WHAT TO EAT AND WHEN: YOUR DAILY EATING PATTERN

Developing your daily eating pattern is easy, and you have unlimited choices to shape your day, as the possible combinations are endless.

Let me show you now one possible daily eating pattern for rapid weight loss. It's my personal favorite because it is so easy to use, and it keeps food coming at me all day long!

## MY FAVORITE RAPID WEIGHT LOSS DAILY EATING PATTERN

**BREAKFAST:** a Revival shake blended with frozen fruit

**MID-MORNING BREAK:** a piece of fruit (e.g. a crisp apple)

**LUNCH:** a chocolate Revival bar and Revival protein chips

**MID-AFTERNOON BREAK:** a salty Revival snack

**DINNER:** a hot entrée with two steaming vegetables

*Alternate:* Revival pasta with two steaming vegetables

**NIGHTTIME SNACK:** bowl of frozen fruit medley

**FLUIDS:** as much calorie-free fluids as desired

**TOTAL FOOD COUNT:** 2 bars/shakes, 5 fruits/veggies, 1 entrée and 2 snacks

*Note:* Any 100-calorie snack can be substituted for a Revival snack!

**TOTAL CALORIE COUNT:** About 1200 calories

When I need to lose weight, I repeat this eating pattern day after day until I have the results I want. Mixing and matching gives you ultimate flexibility so you are never isolated from eating with your family and friends, and the weight maintenance pattern (later in this chapter) has even more choice and flexibility.

I highly recommend you stick with the same daily eating pattern when trying to lose weight to make your diet life simple. Using the same routine every day helps you develop a healthy habit too. As you become more savvy on the diet plan, don't be afraid to mix up your pattern if you want to do so.

To design a different pattern, just grab a sheet of paper or use the simple template found in the *Resources to Rule Your World* section at the back of the book. My nutrition staff can help you develop your plan (just contact us). My online diet management program at **www.RevivalDiet.com** is also a great way to plan your daily eating pattern.

For rapid weight loss, you should drink calorie-free liquids (e.g. water, tea, or diet soda), but you can easily enjoy calorie-containing drinks (e.g. natural fruit juices) as substitutes for a fruit and vegetable serving.

Employ healthy snacks to prevent a tsunami hunger wave from hitting you all at once. Letting too much hunger build up without satisfying it is a guaranteed way to blow up your daily calorie intake with an uncontrolled eating spree.

---

### MOM'S BRIGHT BITE

We are all guilty of having little dieting tricks stuffed up our sleeves that we wrongly use to sneak in a few more unneeded calories. Here's my favorite one:

**WOMAN:** I'd like a triple vanilla ice cream sundae with chocolate syrup, nuts, whipped cream, topped off with a slice of tomato.
**WAITER:** Did I hear you right? Did you say top it off with a slice of tomato?
**WOMAN:** Good heavens, you're right! Forget the tomato—I'm on a diet!

If "sweet abstinence" isn't exactly your cup of tea, then you will love this simple and delicious diet. I've already said, "I do!" for life.

---

Taking a good multivitamin rich in antioxidants during weight loss is very important to protect your body from nutritional deficiencies and to neutralize unhealthy free radicals. The right antioxidants and other newly discovered dietary supplement ingredients can also perfect and protect the appearance of your skin, hair, and nails (read the *Beauty and the Beanstalk* chapter for details).

The daily mental decision to take extra vitamins, minerals, antioxidants, and skin smoothing ingredients is a super easy choice in my mind. Picturing my body exposed to evil (e.g., pollution in the air and free radicals), and without maximum nourishment for my skin, hair, and nails, makes me take a dietary supplement every single day. Make it that simple in your mind, too. *Just take it!*

## THE POWER OF A STRUCTURED EATING PATTERN

Albert Einstein would love this diet because he said, "Everything should be made as simple as possible, but not simpler." Rapid weight loss can't be any easier or healthier. It's very important to understand the power this diet can bring to your life, so I decided to take a few paragraphs to discuss it.

> **FACT:** The simplified structure of this diet—
> using the right delicious foods, including bars and
> shakes—empowers you to bring immediate
> pound-shedding structure to your daily eating pattern.

Protein-packed bars and shakes that satisfy hunger, empower you to make it through the day without "blowing up" your calorie intake from unstructured meals that you have to loosely throw together all of the time. Bars and shakes put you *firmly* in control of your daily colories by acting as the cornerstones of your newly remodeled "house." Say goodbye to the sloppiness of unstructured plans! The protein keeps you feeling fuller longer.

People burn out on unstructured, complicated systems that require too much effort or planning. Long-term results are hard to achieve. Who has time for hundreds of recipes that require you to practically be a full-time gourmet chef? Like a cancer that slowly devours your body, unstructured diets slowly devour your willpower. Most diets are guilty of what I call dietary malpractice because they give us false hope, not long-term results. On the other hand, studies verify that a simplified diet structure empowers you to achieve *beautiful, sustainable results* . . . and that makes me very happy as a medical research doctor. So, if you are hoping for excellent reductions in your gelatinous belly and body fat using this diet, you should be smiling.

Unfortunately, many people believe dietary suffering is required to be healthy: "If it tastes good, it must not be healthy," they say. They have been duped into believing the "No pain, no gain!" philosophy—a diet has to be hard in order to be good.

My philosophy is you have already suffered enough emotionally and physically from your extra pounds. Why would I want to make you suffer further by forcing a complicated diet on you? When I know you would not enjoy it or follow it long-term. I chose to research a plan that was easy for you.

Let's take a quick peak at calories and then learn about the delicious products we can use to lose.

---

### MOM'S BRIGHT BITE

God must really love calories—he made so many of them!

---

## HOW DO THE CALORIES BREAK DOWN ON THIS DIET?

*The Revival Slim & Beautiful Diet* keeps your hunger satisfied while reducing your daily calorie intake to about 1200 calories for rapid weight loss. You will enjoy tons of protein to crush your cravings, so don't worry about feeling hungry. Your calories will vary slightly based on which products you choose to enjoy, but your daily eating pattern makes it simple enough to consistently hit the mark.

## HERE'S HOW THE CALORIES BREAK DOWN

(no M.D. degree required!)

1.  Enjoy 2 to 3 Revival milk protein or soy protein bars and shakes.
    **EQUALS:** 400 – 600 calories
2.  Enjoy 5 servings of fruits and vegetables of your choice.
    **EQUALS:** 400 calories
3.  Enjoy 1 low-calorie meal or pre-packaged entrée of your choice.
    **EQUALS:** 200 – 300 calories

**BONUS SNACKS:** Enjoy 2 Revival snacks substituted for 1 bar or shake.
**EQUALS:** 200 calories (about 100 calories per snack)

**TOTAL CALORIE COUNT:** About 1200 calories

Slow weight loss is better than no weight loss. If you find that 1200 calories per day is simply not enough to keep you happy, then I would recommend increasing your calorie intake to 1400 to 1600 per day by adding in additional food items. You will not lose weight as fast, but you will still be meandering down the hill instead of just stopping dead in your tracks.

## LOSING MORE THAN TWO POUNDS PER WEEK

Working under your healthcare provider's supervision, you can lower your total calorie count to less than 1200 per day and/or increase your physical activity level. It's easy to adjust your daily eating pattern—simply eliminate items (e.g., skip one of the snacks), or keep your entrée calorie count low (i.e., go for 200 calorie entrées instead of 300 calorie entrées). Using these strategies, you and your doctor can lower your total calorie count to around 1000 calories per day or less. I don't recommend eliminating any of the bars or shakes, because they deliver the highest amount of hunger-satisfying, low-glycemic protein to you. Dine wisely with your healthcare provider's help and permission.

---

### MOM'S BRIGHT BITE

Amazing! You hang something in your closet long enough and it shrinks two sizes!

---

## HEY, DAD . . . MOM LOVES IT! . . .
## FOODS TO LOVE AND LOSE

Mom and I understand that people won't stay on a diet or continue to drink, eat, or use a product that they don't absolutely love. That's why taste is our highest priority. Let's listen to Revival-LITES who love the products:

*The Revival bars are absolutely the best! Stop now, no more changes, these are the greatest! The bars melt in your mouth—delicious. I have to lock them up in my desk because my coworkers smell them and want them!*

—K. DEBUSK, NURSE PRACTITIONER

*The shakes taste great. I look forward to them every morning. They're addictive, that's how good they are.*

—F. SPRINGER

*It tastes like a chocolate milkshake, not at all like it is good for me!*

—S. LODGE

*I have been sleeping better. I have more energy, more normal cholesterol levels, and a clearer mind. I feel better than I did when I was thirty! I am now fifty!! Very tasty flavor. I look forward to eating Revival. It's delicious! My skin and hair look better than ever. Thank you so much. Keep those Revival bars coming!*

—L. LONG, Results not typical.[1]

*Revival is awesome. It has been wonderful. The snacks are great. I love the chips. It's like eating junk food, but guess what . . . there's no junk.*

—L. WIGGINS

*Revival helped me to satisfy my chocolate cravings.*

—A.M. DENHUP

Unfortunately, many diet and health product companies have put taste near the bottom of their priority lists. I'm astonished intellectually, and disappointed medically, with diet companies that expect someone who loves, a little too much, great-tasting food (e.g. someone who is fat) to eat a bar that tastes like a cardboard box or drink a shake that tastes like mothballs. Astounding! When I've taste-tested many of these other products, I've thought, "Wow! I could really lose a lot of weight on this product because it tastes so bad I would never eat!" Where do these people and companies come from? Are they from the same planet as us?

Fortunately for everyone (including me) mom is Revival's "Taste-Tester-in-Chief." Trust me, no one is pickier than her when it comes to the taste of food. She's been described more than once as a flavor freak!

She understands good food. I guess because she was cooking meals every day for her entire family by the age of eleven (my grandparents were working on the farm). And, she even won over my dad's heart with her cooking skills.

At the risk of being too dramatic, let me put it this way: if she were a cat, she would be featured in those finicky cat food commercials where our feline friends only dare to eat the moistest, most exquisite cat food. I think you get the point.

Before Revival, we tried every product we could find on the market for her—none were up to her standards. Dad lost count of how many bags of other products had to be taken to the trashcan because of their unbearable taste.

So, mom and I have worked many years to develop new flavors that you won't believe until you taste the proof in our milk protein or soy protein products. You can even have chocolate or your other favorite flavors every single day if you want and still lose weight. Anyone smiling?

## Milk Protein or Soy Protein?

You can choose to enjoy milk-protein-based bars, shakes, and snacks, or soy-protein-based bars, shakes, and snacks, or use both in combination. Mom and I use both for the best variety and full beauty benefits. If you have memories of jiggly-wiggly, bland tofu dancing in your head, fear no evil. I'm a realist, remember. Our new flavor technologies put "joy" into soy, and "marvelous" into milk.

Most Revival products are low-glycemic or "smart-carb," meaning they will not cause a rapid rise in your blood-sugar levels. High blood-sugar levels lead to over-secretion of insulin, which causes some extra blood sugar to be stored as fat.

## Bars and Shakes

Revival bars and shakes come in a large variety of sophisticated, delicious flavors like Chocolate Peanut Haute Couture, Double Chocolate Cover Shot, Peanut Peanut Purr!, Vanilla In Vogue, Chocolate Mint Supermodel, Yogurt Almond Allure, and Chocolate Little Black Dress to just name a few.

How does a thick layer of fine milk chocolate enveloping roasted peanuts, creamy peanut butter, and puffed crisps in a decadent snack bar sound? Or puffed crisps combined with the taste of ripe autumn apples and fresh ground cinnamon finished off with a light frosted glaze of creamy yogurt? And, sweet cocoa in a velvety smooth shake designed to satisfy the most relentless choco-late craving?

Each meticulously formulated bar or shake is packed with 20 grams of milk protein or soy protein, and bone-healthy calcium, and they come in a variety of sweetener choices.

## Snacks, Pasta, and "Coffee"

Revival's crispy protein chips, crunchy sweet and savory soy nuts, and other nutritious snacks are the perfect cure for between-meal and late-night snack-ing urges. Plus, they give you an energy-boosting pick-me-up for mid-morn-ing or mid-afternoon slumps.

Our delicious protein-packed chips are baked to crispy perfection then generously flavored with a variety of seasoning for a taste that is unforget-table. You will want to eat a lot more than just one, but it is okay because they are so healthy!

Our protein-packed pasta offers the same authentic flavor and texture of Old World pasta, but with twice the protein and 25 percent fewer carbs than regular pasta.

Revival's crunchy, fresh-roasted soy nuts seasoned to perfection or coated with chocolate or yogurt satisfy your salty, sweet, and crunchy hunger crav-ings. We even have soy-based "coffee" made from fresh roasted soy nuts.

Like mom says, the taste of Revival products will make you "purrrrrrr!" You will find lots to love with Revival, and lots less of your body fat. We are constantly developing new products, so check with us for the latest flavors and variety.

If you want to get a head start on your beauty diet goals while you finish reading this book, contact my friendly nutrition staff for expert advice at **1-800-REVIVAL** (1-800-738-4825), **www.RevivalDiet.com**, or **Nutrition@RevivalDiet.com**.

It's super easy to start because they will help you select the perfect *Revival Slim and Beautiful Diet* package containing all the exact products you need to jumpstart your beauty diet results.

Customers love the savings and convenience of Revival's auto-delivery program. Doubt our taste in food? Free samples are available, with only a small shipping and handling fee. Great variety packs are also available. We even have an antioxidant-rich complete beauty vitamin to perfect and protect the appearance of your skin, hair, and nails while supplying you with all the vitamins and minerals needed for healthy weight loss.

## MOM'S BRIGHT BITE

Don't you just love those mirrors? Read this cute, but oh-so-true, poem!

Mirror, mirror on the wall, do you have to tell it all?
Where do you get the glaring right, to make my clothes look just
   too tight?
I think I'm fine, but I can see, you won't cooperate with me.
The way you let the shadows play, you'd think my hair was getting gray!
What's that, you say? A double chin? No, that's the way the light
   comes in;
If you persist in peering so, you'll confiscate my facial glow,
And then if you're not hanging straight, you'll tell me next I'm
   gaining weight;
I'm really quite upset with you, for giving this distorted view;
I hate you being smug and wise; Oh, look what's happened to my
   thighs!
I warn you now, O mirrored wall, since we're not on speaking terms at all,
If I look like this in my new jeans, you'll find yourself in smithereens!

—ANONYMOUS

Because of our medical research, all of Revival's "mom-approved" products come with a 100 percent satisfaction and great-taste guarantee.

Your purchase of Revival products helps feed hungry boys and girls worldwide. You can learn more at **www.RevivalDiet.com/Children**.

## HUNGER DOESN'T HAVE A PRAYER
## AGAINST THE POWER OF PROTEIN!†

Chase away hunger by eating more protein! This protein-packed diet will help you feel fuller longer by sending "I'm full" messages from your stomach to your brain. Help for your urge to splurge is on its way with typically 50 to 75 grams of protein per day on this plan (40 to 60 daily grams from Revival bars and shakes).

## TELL FAT TO "MOOOOOOVE AWAY" WITH MILK PROTEIN!

High-quality, easily-digested milk proteins include casein and whey, which provide all the essential "amino acids" (building blocks for our bodies) required for proper human nutrition. Research suggests that milk proteins have a variety of benefits for human health, including fitness, weight management, cardiovascular health, normal bone health support, and antioxidant support. Milk protein is rich in branched-chain amino acids that can be burned to produce energy and used to build more calorie-burning lean muscle mass.

## "SHAKE IT UP, BABY!" AND SHAKE OUT
## THE FAT WITH SOY PROTEIN!

Before Revival, soy protein used to come in only four flavors: chalky, bland, icky, and worse than icky! But new flavoring technologies have

---

†These statements have not been evaluated by the Food and Drug Administration. Revival is not intended to diagnose, treat, cure, or prevent any disease.

eliminated the traditional soy taste, making Revival nutritious and delicious.

Revival's soy protein is affectionately called, "The Sexiest Protein on the Planet" because it is the only protein clinically proven for weight loss *and* better skin, hair, and nails.

Interestingly, soy is the only vegetable that supplies a complete source of high-quality, easily digested protein rich in all of the essential amino acids needed for building lean muscle mass and supporting normal human growth and development. Like milk protein, soy protein is rich in "branched-chain amino acids" for an energy source and promotion of calorie-burning lean muscle mass. Soy is also the only vegetable that naturally contains more protein than carbohydrates!

In addition to regular Revival soy-protein-based products, "naturally concentrated" Revival bars and shakes are designed to supplement your diet with soy antioxidants. Using our patented process, we harvest the concentrated goodness from the antioxidant-rich soybean heart. Just one naturally concentrated bar or shake supplement contains the same amount of soy antioxidants found in 6 cups of a typical soymilk, thus making it easy to enjoy the full soy antioxidant benefits for your skin, hair, nails, and body. For the intellectually curious, soy's antioxidants are called "isoflavones."

With the added power of Revival's natural concentration, a separate Revival study (detailed in the *Beauty and the Beanstalk* chapter) shows you can significantly rejuvenate the appearance of your skin, hair, and nails from the inside out. Individual results vary, but you'll see the visible signs of aging diminish with smoother-looking skin and a softer glow. You'll also notice your hair growing longer and silkier, just like my mom's beautiful midlife mane. And you may be able to skip those appointments for artificial nails, as your own grow stronger.

It's easy to include a naturally concentrated Revival bar or shake dietary supplement as part your daily eating pattern on either the milk-protein-based diet or soy-protein-based diet.

## TIME FOR A "FRUIT AND VEGGIE MAKEOVER" WITH THE LITTLE GREEN GIANTS . . . AND RED AND ORANGE AND YELLOW AND PURPLE AND BLUE GIANTS!

A small amount of daily fruits and vegetables can produce giant success. There is gold at the end of the rainbow. In other words, eat several colors of fruit and veggies for the best results and a healthy skin glow. Aim for at least five servings of three or more colors per day. Make variety the spice of your success.

---

### MOM'S BRIGHT BITE

Q:  How do you know carrots are good for your eyes?

A:  You never see a rabbit wearing glasses!

---

## FRESH VERSUS FROZEN VERSUS CANNED VERSUS DRIED?

The answer is: Use whatever is the most convenient for you (which is usually a blend of all). Today's "fresh-frozen" technology preserves every drop of goodness in fruits and vegetables picked at the peak of ripeness, flavor, and nutritional content. Your frozen grocery aisle has an amazing selection of fresh-frozen veggies that make fabulous in-the-box low-calorie additions to any meal or snack time. Just pop them in the microwave and they emerge hot and steamy—so yummy and wholesome! Frozen fruits, particularly blends containing peaches, mango, grapes, pineapple, and cantaloupe, or even just frozen grapes (buy fresh, rinse, and throw into the freezer), are our favorites. Canned or dried fruits and vegetables are another option with lots of great-tasting variety.

By the way, carrots *are* great for your eyes and skin because they are rich in the vitamin-A precursor beta-carotene. But, no, ketchup is *not* a vegetable.

Someone once said to me, "Any vegetable tastes great if you put enough butter and salt on it—even brussel sprouts!" I'll give you a big fat "no" on that one, too. Use a cholesterol-lowering spread instead and limit your salt intake (excessive salt is linked to stomach cancer). Rule: moderation equals minimization of your waistline.

---

## MOM'S BRIGHT BITE

Q: Why did the tomato blush?
A: He saw the salad dressing!

One of my favorite ways to enjoy tomatoes is to slice them, then bake slowly (200 degrees for several hours) coated with basil, olive oil, pepper and salt. I can feel the extra beauty benefits of the olive oil in my skin, hair, and nails.

---

Don't blow your calorie count through the unscrupulous use of fat-laden dressings. Tomatoes are great for better skin color appearance due to their rich concentration of a red-colored antioxidant called lycopene. As lycopene content decreases in our skin with age, we become pale and washed out—we lose our "redness." Eating tomatoes can put some pink back into our skin.

---

## MOM'S BRIGHT BITE

Q: Why did the potato go to the beach?
A: Because he wanted to get baked.

When craving potatoes, reach for the sweets! Sweet potatoes are especially nutritious and delicious. Try slicing them thin and baking for kid-approved snacks.

Baked potatoes in moderation are okay, and you can still look great at the beach if you eat them sparingly. Of course, don't bake *yourself*. Limit sun exposure during peak hours and wear sunscreen to block collagen-destroying sun rays.

## MOM'S BRIGHT BITE

Q: How do you make a strawberry shake?
A: Put it in the refrigerator!

Q: What did the banana say to the doctor?
A: I'm not peeling very well!

Make your kids or grandkids think you are "cool" by sharing these fruit and veggie jokes with them! They are a great way to start educating kids about better nutrition. Strawberries are the first fruit to ripen in the spring, so to me they are a low-calorie symbol of a new day and a new start. Try lengthy slices of banana coated with organic crunchy peanut butter for your nighttime snack.

It's easy and delicious to blend frozen fruits into Revival shakes for extra antioxidants. My favorites are adding frozen strawberries or a frozen banana to a Revival chocolate shake. Oh, but make sure you peel the banana before freezing it (I learned the hard way). Frozen peaches, frozen blueberries, or fresh orange juice are delicious in a Revival vanilla shake. The extra vitamin C and antioxidants in fruits are excellent for better-looking skin.

---

### MOM'S BRIGHT BITE

Q What did Baby Corn ask Mama Corn?
A: Where's Pop Corn?

I know, you are thinking "corny," but fresh-popped popcorn lightly salted with a cholesterol-lowering spread is one of my favorite ways to share a healthy snack with my husband while we watch a great movie.

---

Low-fat popcorn makes a great fiber-rich snack. Zipped bags full of popcorn and sliced apples make great traveling buddies. I bet you thought I was going to say, "An apple a day keeps the doctor away."

---

### MOM'S BRIGHT BITE

Sorry, Charlie . . . it grieves me to tell you that chocolate-covered raisins, cherries, and strawberries do not count as fruits!

---

If more specific fruit and veggie recommendations would be helpful for you, please visit **www.RevivalDiet.com**, or contact my nutrition staff at 1-800-REVIVAL (1-800-738-4825) or **Nutrition@RevivalDiet.com**.

## MAKE YOUR ENTICING ENTRANCE WITH ENTRÉES!

With so many delicious new pre-packaged fresh and frozen entrée options emerging regularly, I want to make sure you hear what we have to say about the latest and greatest products. Many of these entrées can be found in your local grocery's frozen foods aisle. My nutrition staff can recommend specific entrée brands and products that taste fabulous while fitting perfectly into the pants of this diet plan, typically with 15 or more grams of protein, 200 to 300 calories, and low levels of bad fats.

Why use entrées? Pre-packaged entrées are excellent for busy dieters because delicious meals can be prepared in only a few minutes in a microwave. New food technologies have produced tons of extremely tasty options high in protein and low in fat and calories.

Prepackaged entrées are also excellent "teachers" about proper portion sizes. When you learn the size of a 200 to 300 calorie entrée, you will have a better idea of how much you should eat the next time you go to a restaurant. Today's "Runaway Restaurants" are killing us with their hugely hazardous serving sizes that make us more huggable but a lot less healthy. All of our moms used to yell across the table at us, "Clean your plate!" Most of us still feel guilty as adults because we were truthfully told that starving kids around the world would gladly finish our dinner if given the opportunity. Our moms *were* right at the time that we should clean our plates, because portion sizes were much smaller then. But, guess what? Great increases in "normal" portion sizes over the past thirty years have led to great increases in our "normal" waistlines. We have to reevaluate the rules and take action!

The best strategy for portion control is simply to not put so much food on our plates in the first place (and it doesn't take Albert Einstein to figure this one out). Once the food is on the plate, we feel obligated to eat it. We feel we *have* to finish the large mountain of mashed potatoes. So, when it comes to portion control, an "ounce of prevention" is worth pounds and pounds of cure. Prevent your guilt to get rid of your gut.

---

### MOM'S BRIGHT BITE

**WOMAN TO WAITER:** "Sir, *what* is that fly doing in my soup?"
**WAITER:** "Ma'am, it looks like the backstroke!"

Smaller portions will stop us from dying like flies!

---

Wondering how to start reducing your current portion size? Obviously if you are overweight the portion size you currently are eating isn't working out for you. So, using the current portion size as a reference, reduce the amount of food on your plate by one quarter (25 percent) to start. Over time, you will probably find that you can reduce your current amount by 33 percent to 50 percent without feeling hungry, particularly if you slow down while eating and savor each bite. Mimic what you see with the entrées—typically a small portion of lean meat (skinless chicken, lean beef, or other meat with the fat trimmed off), a small portion of starch (such as potato or rice), and a small portion of veggies. Just use the brain you were created to use.

Enjoyed properly, entrées and sensible meals help you make a great entrance to this eating plan! They also help you make a great entrance into a smaller dress or pants' size.

For specific entrée recommendations, visit **www.RevivalDiet.com**, or contact my Nutrition Staff at **1-800-REVIVAL** (1-800-738-4825) or **Nutrition@RevivalDiet.com**.

## DOCTOR-PRESCRIBED SHOPPING FOR THE PHYSICAL ACTIVITY PLAN?

You've learned the super simple eating plan. The physical activity plan is just as simple. Shopping for new walking shoes is an important part of achieving amazing results on this diet. Buy several pairs and make sure someone who loves you pays for them—it's a doctor-approved expense that's essential to help you achieve the great weight loss results seen in the Revival clinical trial.

---

**FACT:** Walking to help burn calories, boost your metabolism, and elevate your mood are doctor's orders!

---

Do you really feel you should sit around on your couch all day reading diet books? Couch potatoes quickly become rotten vegetables. Had overeating combined with lack of physical activity been a large problem during Benjamin Franklin's time, I'm sure he would have added "couch potatoes" to his famous statement, "Fish and visitors smell after three days."

Walking is pain-free, fun, and relaxing, so there is absolutely no excuse for being a couch potato (complaining about walking does not help you burn any extra calories). Walking also gives you time to think, pray, or meditate about your day while listening to your favorite energizing music.

---

### MOM'S BRIGHT BITE

You know it is time to start walking regularly when you start believing, "If God really wanted me to touch my toes, He would have put them near my knees!"

---

## INACTIVITY EQUALS INGRATITUDE

Being inactive on purpose is shameful. Mom and I both have been guilty of inactivity in the past. Do you know how many people would give anything to have the ability to walk for the first time, or to walk again? If we believe every day is truly a gift, then let's make actual walking just as important as our figurative walking down the diet hill.

We were simply not designed to be motionless. It just isn't right! Burning an extra 2500 or more calories per week is the physical activity goal for great weight loss results based on what dieters in the Revival study burned weekly. This can be accomplished by walking briskly thirty to forty-five minutes per day (which can be divided into several ten-to-fifteen-minute power walks throughout the day) for six days per week. Making a commitment to physical activity six days per week will remind you of the importance of faithfully following the eating plan.

If you "don't have enough time" to be physically active, I recommend taking immediate steps to rearrange your life—your health obviously is not near the top of your priority list where it should be. In the meantime, using a stationary bike or treadmill for twenty to thirty minutes six times per week is an adequate substitute that requires less time.

Grab a pal, a puppy, or an iPod to listen to your favorite tunes—whatever it takes to start walking! It will help make you sparkle while taking the pounds off. If you need daily motivation to help you, join my online diet management program at **www.RevivalDiet.com**, or contact my nutrition staff for specific recommendations on at-home walking programs with video coaching to motivate you.

### That's it for the physical activity plan!

Can you lose weight just by dieting without the physical activity? Of course you can, but I'm not sure why anyone dreaming of a beautiful new body and life they love would want to miss out on the uplifting energy and accelerated weight loss results from physical activity. Skipping the physical activity part of this plan is a really bad idea. Period. You won't achieve the incredible results found in the Revival diet study in just sixteen weeks, and you definitely won't be as proud of yourself as you should be.

Back to the important part—shopping! Make sure your new walking shoes have great arch support to protect your feet. Walking at the local shopping mall is great exercise (and a free indoor track for rainy days), so shop 'til you drop!

New walking shoes: $60

Cute new walking outfit: $50

Bottle of ice-cold water: $2

Burning calories, boosting metabolism, and elevating mood:
Priceless . . .

---

### MOM'S BRIGHT BITE

Walking is a great way to stay in shape and live longer. My mother started walking when she was sixty. She's ninety now and we have no idea where she is!

---

## WEIGHT MAINTENANCE USING THE REVIVAL SLIM AND BEAUTIFUL DIET

Once you have dropped all of the gelatinous baggage you desired to lose, or if you simply want to take a day or more off from losing weight, you can easily switch to a weight-maintenance pace.

Yes, I just gave you permission to take a break from this diet when you need it. Everyone needs a break from time to time. Being *persistent* over time using this diet is much more important than unrealistic *perfection*. Persistence is persevering in spite of opposition, obstacles, and discouragement. Persistently using this diet plan, despite all the obstacles you face, will consistently cause you to lose weight and become more beautiful.

For weight maintenance, the *Revival Slim and Beautiful Diet* keeps your daily calorie intake at about 1800 to 2000 calories (that's a lot of extra food and snacks you get to enjoy compared to the rapid weight loss plan!)

## HOW TO MAINTAIN YOUR WEIGHT

Here's how a weight maintenance day would look:

1. Enjoy 1 to 2 Revival milk protein or soy protein bars and shakes.
   **EQUALS** 200 – 400 calories.
2. Enjoy 5 servings of fruits and vegetables of your choice.
   **EQUALS** 400 calories.
3. Enjoy 2 low-calorie meals or pre-packaged entrées OR
   1 sensible meal.
   **EQUALS** 400 – 800 calories.

**BONUS SNACKS:** Enjoy 2 to 4 Revival snacks (or any 100-calorie snack)
**EQUALS** 200 – 400 calories.

**TOTAL CALORIE COUNT:** About 1800 – 2000 calories

Most people will find their "sweet spot" for weight maintenance between 1800 and 2000 calories per day. However, if you find yourself regaining weight on 1800 to 2000 calories per day, make a slight adjustment to reduce calories by cutting out a snack or decreasing the calorie content of an entrée. You have the power to change it. You can adjust your maintenance pattern just like your rapid weight loss pattern.

Are you sure you can eat this much? Check out all of the food you get to constantly enjoy throughout the day during weight maintenance:

## MY FAVORITE WEIGHT MAINTENANCE DAILY EATING PATTERN

**BREAKFAST:** a Revival shake blended with frozen fruit

**MID-MORNING BREAK:** a piece of fruit and Revival protein chips

**LUNCH:** a hot entrée with a steaming vegetable

**MID-AFTERNOON BREAK:** a chocolate Revival bar and salty snack

**DINNER:** a hot entrée with two steaming vegetables

*Alternate:* Revival pasta with two steaming vegetables

**NIGHTTIME SNACK:** a sweet Revival snack and salty snack

**FLUIDS:** as much calorie-free fluids as desired

**TOTAL FOOD COUNT:** 2 bars/shakes, 5 fruits/veggies, 2 entrées, and 4 snacks

*Note:* Any 100-calorie snack can be substituted for a Revival snack!

**TOTAL CALORIE COUNT:** About 1800 – 2000 calories

You can design your own maintenance pattern using a sheet of paper or the simple template found in the *Resources to Rule Your World* section.

P.S. No one gave you permission to stop being physically active!

## ARE YOU READY TO MAKE YOUR RESERVATIONS?

You will feel incredibly empowered and proud when you finally take control of your weight and beauty. *Thousands* of Revival-LITES are living a life they love. If you are really, really ready to join them, call **1-800-REVIVAL** or visit **www.RevivalDiet.com** to make reservations for your dream vacation far, far away from ugly, gelatinous fat. In the meantime, let's go crazy about becoming slim and beautiful!

## LET'S GO CRAZY ABOUT DIET SUCCESS!

I'm excited in the coming chapters to share more detailed medical research on the remarkable health benefits of this diet, particularly gorgeous skin, hair, and nails. So, keep your diet boots made for walking on, but let's also put on our thinking caps for the next chapter.

It's time we get into great psychological shape for dieting success. Psychological shape? Here's what I mean: A proper mental mindset will produce maximum weight loss and beauty results. In other words, a smarter mind equals a slimmer body.

My "Ten Psychological Commandments of Permanent Weight Loss" in the next chapter will help you reign sovereign over fat.

Let's go!

## CHAPTER 3

# The Ten Psychological Commandments of Permanent Weight Loss

*Inside me there's a thin person struggling to get out, but I can usually sedate her with four or five cupcakes.*
—ANONYMOUS

*Most folks are as happy as they make up their minds to be.*
—ABRAHAM LINCOLN

*After starting Revival, I noticed a difference in my overall energy level. My weight started out at 184 pounds and has now dropped to 150 pounds (a 34-pound drop), and I am continuing to lose! My plan is to stay on Revival for the rest of my life. I have not only incorporated Revival shakes into my daily routine, but I love the bars for on the go. I can't imagine living today without my Revival. It is a wonderful boost to my morning. It just completely has changed my life for the good. Without all the extra pounds, I am more confident, energetic, and excited about being forty-seven! I am probably in the best shape of my life, thanks to Revival.*

—J. SITEK, Results not typical.[†]

---

[†]Results not typical, but included to motivate you. Individual results vary. You must follow the calorie-restricted diet plan, physical activity plan, and dietary supplement regimens presented in this book if you hope to achieve great weight loss, beauty, and health results. see *Introduction* and specific studies presented in this book for typical results. These statements have not been evaluated by the Food and Drug Administration. Revival is not intended to diagnose, treat, cure, or prevent any disease.

I recommend you read and reread this chapter frequently. It is the most important chapter in the book for winning our "slim and beautiful" nutritional war. Ironically, this chapter has nothing to do with clinically–proven nutrition, but it does have everything to do with mentally–proven determination for permanent weight loss.

After meeting my mom and me, people often comment on how well we balance each other. Though a strong businesswoman, Mom has also been graced with a tender heart and lots of empathy! She's writing this book with me to keep a good balance of understanding counselor to go with my "Just Do It!" medical research style, but I have to warn you for the duration of this chapter, mom is out of the room.

My truthfulness may not only change your waistline, but could save your life. I hope this chapter really opens your eyes to the truth, permanently.

**FACT:** I am passionate about your health and sometimes that means I am tough, especially on any excuse that is making you fat and killing you!

I want to make sure you are losing weight for all of the right reasons, reasons that will help you keep the weight off permanently. So here's my Ten Psychological Commandments for making your mind smarter so your body is slimmer. No holds barred: the weight stops here!

So, just relax on the psychological diet couch while we have a session on the deeper meanings of dieting. This is the only time you are allowed to be a couch potato with my blessing, so try to enjoy it!

**FACT:** If we are trying to lose weight only to look better in a bathing suit, we are headed toward an ugly failure.

Millions fail to keep the pounds off because they are trying to lose weight for all the wrong reasons. The good news is that we can train our minds to choose powerful, right reasons to lose the fat and keep it off, permanently.

One of my favorite sayings is, "Persistence always dominates." Constantly pressing onward to make our dreams a reality will make them happen. Note that I said "persistence," not "perfection." None of us are perfect.

We all have our "saint days" and "sinner days" when it comes to dieting, but the key is to be persistent. If we persist in fighting the good fight by taking the following commandments to heart, it will lead to *consistently* winning in the nutritional war. We will dominate our fat and wrinkles.

## 1. Thou shalt not worship food as your god.

Food was designed to serve us—not to make us ugly and fat and then kill us! We should never put food before our health, happiness, and beauty. When we are overeating, we are placing our minds and bodies in the direct path of disease and death. The impact is inevitable, and the fall-out of such an ugly crash affects not only you, but all who love you.

Food should serve us with health-building nourishment, giving us energy and great-looking skin, hair, and nails that we are proud to possess. Are we serving food that is making us fat, ugly, and disease-prone instead? If you are, it should make you downright mad and disgusted at the situation. Show a little R-E-S-P-E-C-T for your body and your mind by not letting food disrespect your beauty and health.

I've already made up my mind to *never* let food dominate my life and my health (where I end up serving the Almighty Fork and Plate)—but I've chosen to have food be my servant, where I'm in control, using it for my higher good.

**FACT:** We can use food to beautify us, instead of betraying us. Working together with this clinically proven plan, we are going to create a beautiful new work of art: you!

Outward changes start with deep inward convictions. You can choose to stop worshipping food right now by taking over the reins. Just say "no."

## 2. Thou shalt not worship a false image.

A false image is an idol that is worshipped. Don't be fooled into worshipping a false image—a body that can only be achieved with the help of extreme plastic surgery and digital photo airbrushing by the beauty and fashion industry. You will never be happy if you pursue such false, superhuman images.

Warped perceptions of our physical appearance are created from the Barbie-type, airbrushed images that surround us everyday. With these unrealistic expectations, it is no wonder so many people are dissatisfied with their bodies, self-conscious, and incapable of appreciating basic good health. This goes especially for women—four out of five females are unhappy with their bodies. The consequences: teenage girls tormented with self-scrutiny, pregnant women deprived of essential nourishment in order to limit weight gain, and the new prevalence of eating disorders among women in midlife.

Even pre-teen girls in America grow up with Barbie dolls, playing out scenes for what their adult lives could be. According to *Marie Claire* magazine, if Barbie were a real woman, she would be seven-foot-two and possess these unlikely measurements: 40-inch bust, 22-inch waist, and 36-inch hips!

Are we allowing our celebrity-obsessed culture to torture our minds (and checkbooks) with impossible idols, instead of maintaining a realistic, beautiful, and healthy body image? It should make us angry enough to change our thoughts and actions! It is critical that we develop a crystal-clear picture of a realistic, beautiful, and healthy body in our mind's eye.

Why is it important to visualize a realistic, perfect body? Because doing so will force us to make a win-or-lose decision with every single meal or snack. We empower ourselves to choose whether or not that extra cookie or fatty bite is really worth wrecking our dreams and health.

Let's take some time right now to visualize the perfect body clearly. Smile while you are doing this! I want you to focus on clearly seeing the *exact* beautiful body that you want to have:

- See softer, sexier skin with diminished wrinkles and discoloration.
- See silkier hair and stronger, longer nails.
- See leaner arms with a trimmer stomach and smaller waistline.

Picture it in your mind.

- See a smaller, firmer *gluteus maximus* that isn't sagging.
- See leaner, toner legs with a tighter skin appearance.

Take some serious time to imagine your beautiful unique self, only leaner, softer, and more beautiful . . . Do you like what you see?

Now, we're really going to put your imagination in hyperdrive—going deep within your body to imagine what you can't see but yet is vital to a long, satisfying life:

- See a healthier brain, heart, circulation system, digestive tract, kidneys, and liver.
- Feel the weight taken off your joints.
- Feel more energy ready to meet and beat the challenges in life.

Take a moment and really feel it.

- Feel a spring in your step with the urge to move.
- See a glow in your eyes and a smile on your face.
- Feel the comfort and satisfaction of total body beauty and wellness.

Now see a life that you and your family love, full of good health, physical activity, and great memories.

I want you to put down this book for a few minutes and see this clearly in your mind. Can you see the metamorphosis taking place? I can. Can you feel the positive changes taking place? I can feel them. We can choose to have the beautiful body and energized life that we have visualized. This is empowerment!

I'm always amazed to see someone's shock when they realize for the very first time that their mind is actually master over their body. The only reason we won't win the war on ugly fat and wrinkles is if we don't consciously force our minds to make win-or-lose decisions about eating.

How can we force our minds to make the right eating decisions? Every single time we start to eat or drink, we have to visualize our perfect body image and ask, "Will this food or drink nourish and beautify my body, or will it pour ugly gelatinous fat, sugar, and chemicals into it?" This forces us to decide whether or not that extra bite or sip is really more valuable to us than our perfect bodies and being with our families.

Will we always choose the "win" decision? Of course not! We are all human, but remember that *persistence always dominates*. If we make win decisions consistently over time, we take steps down the right path to our perfect bodies.

Defeat is only temporary until the next win-or-lose decision. If we make the wrong decision we have to immediately decide to make the right decision the next time.

We will refuse to let small, temporary defeats spiral out of control and derail our walk. Let's not be guilty of the Perfectionist Dieter's Creed: "If I fall off my diet, I've failed, and therefore I am a total failure . . . and therefore, I might as well eat this entire pint of ice cream and anything else I find calling my name from the recesses of the fridge. I am a diet sinner and an unworthy worm. Therefore I will eat everything in sight."

We've all been at this point in the past, but let's refuse to go there in the future. Our inner psychological change gives us the power to say no to spiraling out of control. We will walk the line over time together.

Our new beautiful bodies are only the outward sign of a true inward change. In the *Your Daily Diet Devotions* chapter, mom and I have included testimonies from Revival customers who are living a life they love by making their dreams reality. You can draw strength from reading several of the testimonials daily—a "daily diet devotion" to uplift and motivate you. Reading the testimonials inspires me to work harder on my research and on my own health.

## 3. Thou shalt not murder.

"Got fat?" If you do, fat has you too—by the throat! Can you feel fat choking you?

Fat kills. Let me spell it out clearly: F-A-T  K-I-L-L-S. Being fat is like holding a lit stick of dynamite in your mouth. It's only a matter of time before it blows your health and dreams to bits.

More than thirty diseases result from excessive fat, including horrific ones like breast cancer, ovarian cancer, diabetes, stroke, and heart disease. Sudden death by heart attack is not an admirable way to die, particularly when you don't get to say goodbye to your loved ones. Studies even show that excessive fat may even make certain cancers more aggressive.

> **FACT:** Fat is a felon—guilty of millions of murders.

Sure, your eating habits may be killing you, but are they also killing your family? I see a day coming when parents may be prosecuted for creating overweight children! Parents are physically abusing their kids when they cause them to become fat, because it predisposes the kids to so many awful diseases.

My dad said something profound to me: "Kids are the only family members that make you feel like royalty every time they see you." My point is that putting precious children in harm's way (which includes smoking around them) is never acceptable. Coupled with the emotional abuse that fat kids suffer from peers, it can be a deadly combination.

It's simple: we can choose to dig our graves with our forks, or we can choose to protect ourselves and families.

To force my mind to make the right decision, I imagine drowning inside of a supersized cake. The frosting smothers me as I struggle to gasp for air— I feel the panic in my lungs! It may sound silly, but it works. And we might as well choke to death on cake frosting if our eating is slowly killing our bodies anyway.

## 4. Thou shalt not steal.

Would you trade your child for a cookie? Is overeating more valuable than your family time? Is being fat more important to you than your friends?

---

**FACT:** We have a critical psychological decision to remake at the start of every day. Do we choose to walk towards a great-looking and long-lived body today, or towards a saggy, fatigued, ugly, and short-lived life? Do we choose to die to our old selves daily, or do we choose to just die?

---

We are being selfish when we place pleasure from overeating before our families and loved ones. Here's why: When we choose to destroy our health and energy, it will eventually kill or debilitate us, therefore we steal valuable time away our families and friends. Do we choose a great life with our children and grandchildren, or do we choose to be a bedridden, financial and emotional burden on them?

We have to make this choice every day.

Irresponsible food and restaurant companies are literally profiting off your disability and death. Will you choose to continue helping them profit from your suffering?

Here's a better question: Can you hear your children saying, "Don't eat so much Mommy and Daddy. I don't want you to die and go away. I need you here"?

Make sure you hear them speaking to you every time you are making a win-or-lose decision over those extra calories. Choose to not let the Fat Fire burn your house down with you and your family in it. Only you can prevent Fat Fires. Remember what you were taught in elementary school to do if you are on fire: Stop, drop the roll!

## 5. Thou shalt not covet.

Is the envy of someone else's body hindering the success of our own *realistic* weight loss goals? Trying to look like celebrities can cripple us psychologically. Why? Because unrealistic, unachievable goals lead to discouragement, which then leads to failure!

Today's pop culture is obsessed with weight. Television shows focus on radical body makeovers and weight loss challenges while tabloids are teeming with photographs that glamorize emaciated celebrities. At the same time, however, headlines pose the question, "Are They too Skinny?" The result—we are consumed with looking good and less concerned about overall health and well-being.

The grass is not always greener or *leaner* on the other side of the fence, whether you are famous or French.

French women don't get fat . . . or do they? If I were to ask you to imagine a French woman in your mind, what would she look like? I bet you are picturing a slender woman, lounging at an outdoor café with a cigarette (hopefully not with her children) and an espresso. Well, recent research has revealed that French women may not be as sexy and svelte as we imagine. About 41 percent of French people are overweight, and this number is growing each year.

We can't let smoke and mirrors warp our perception of reality. Let's keep it real by choosing to focus on healthy, realistic goals.

> **FACT:** Setting a realistic, achievable *first* weight loss
> goal is critical to our success, because it keeps us
> psychologically content. After we achieve the first goal,
> we can then set a new goal that is even better!
> We can and will repeat this over and over.

Understand what I'm saying? Choose a weight loss goal that you know you can achieve. Maybe your first goal is to lose 5 pounds. Let's lose those

5 pounds then set a new, better goal. Using this stepped approach is a powerful psychological tool for long-term weight loss.

Think about walking down a staircase. It would be silly, dangerous, and scary to try to jump all the way to the bottom, or to even try stepping down more than one step at a time. Instead, we systematically take the first step downward followed by a second step downward and so on. This makes walking down simple and safe.

Setting a first goal that you know is impossible will destroy your success and scare you. We humans are more likely to stay motivated if we are able to meet our goal in a fairly short amount of time. So it is better to set small, sequential, achievable goals.

Make sure you reward yourself in some small way at each phase, but not with a banana split. Instead get a makeover with friends! Take a day off to yourself to do anything you want to do all day long—sleep in, watch a movie, go shopping or golfing or to a sports or music event. Or, drive to a beautiful place and read a great book.

Celebrating with friends who have also reached their goal is the best calorie-free treat in life.

Let's choose to take small steps—or in our case, smaller bites—together toward our ultimate goals.

## 6. Thou shalt not cheat against thy confidence and self-esteem.

Has prior diet cheating or diet failure harmed your self-esteem? Failed dieting cycles can hurt something much more important than our wallets—it can hurt our self-respect and confidence to succeed.

Many people spend money on diet programs that falsely guarantee rapid weight loss. These devilish diets use false marketing claims and untested plans to give us false hope. We hungrily try to deprive ourselves of food on these diets against our own common sense. Then we feel guilty and humiliated because we've either cheated on the diet, or strictly followed directions to only achieve minimal results.

Sound familiar?

This dieting pattern produces emotional damage in our confidence to succeed. We start doubting if we will ever be able to look beautiful and fit. Our self-esteem darkens.

---

**FACT:** Small successes are the best medicine to start healing injured confidence and self-esteem. We will rebuild our self-respect and confidence better than ever. How? Winning the small battles over and over by taking the small steps.

---

If you have fallen on your face because you trusted in one of these false hopes, you are not alone! Millions of dieters have unwittingly trusted in unattainable promises, only to fail and suffer the psychological consequences. There is one word to describe companies claiming 10 pounds of permanent weight loss in one weekend: liars.

Our nutritional war will be won inch by inch. Every small win will help us build more confidence to win the next victory. To the victor goes the spoils—a beautiful and healthy body living a life that can be loved. As each inch is conquered, our waistlines will continue to shrink.

Choose to rebuild your self-esteem, confidence, and health by winning the small battles!

## 7. Thou shalt not lie.

Are we lying to ourselves about the true cause of our overeating? Are there insidious reasons behind our eating addictions that we are failing to recognize? Is stress, depression, or frustration negatively impacting our dietary choices?

Everyone knows that eating and our emotions are intertwined. We don't have to have endless research studies or scientific debates to know it's the truth. We all look to food for comfort, energy, happiness, and more.

**FACT:** We need to discover the cause of our overeating
so we can effectively fight it. We have to know
what the the enemy is before we can defeat it!
Understanding why and when we overeat will help us win.

Chemical messengers in our brain (called "neurotransmitters") respond to food intake by affecting our emotions, cravings, and appetites. For example, the messenger *serotonin* controls feelings of satisfaction and happiness. Low levels of serotonin are associated with depression, decreased energy, and increased appetite. Stress can deplete serotonin, which may account for why we have food cravings when we are experiencing tense or difficult times in our lives.

People who are sad or fatigued may crave chocolate. The sugar and fat combination from chocolate is believed to increase serotonin and endorphin levels. Many parents give their child candy to soothe an injury or sadness. This may cause the child to mentally associate candy with comfort, even into adulthood.

A recent study found that people's eating patterns altered based on their mood. While not set in stone, the results are interesting (this is one of the reasons that I've created healthy Revival products that satisfy cravings for sweet, salty, and crunchy foods):

- Stressed: salty foods like crisps and soy sauce
- In need of comfort: ice cream
- Sad: sugary foods and caffeine
- Sexually frustrated: pretzels, breads, and crackers
- Lonely: rice and pasta

How do we identify overeating caused by emotions? Most people can discover their triggers simply by taking some quiet time to analyze it mentally. An important question to ask yourself is, "Under what mental condition am

I most likely to overeat?" Most of us already know what our weaknesses are. My most vulnerable situations are caused by stress, particularly if I'm working late at night. It's easy to want to toss a pizza in the oven or munch on sour candies. If you can't figure it out just by thinking about it, keep a simple food diary for a week by writing down what foods are consumed at what time, and how you were feeling at the time.

You may discover that there is not an emotional trigger related to your eating, but that is still very valuable information to know! It means your cause of overeating is simply physical hunger. You can take steps with the *Revival Slim and Beautiful Diet* to satisfy your hunger without blowing up your calorie consumption.

And if you routinely crave a specific food that is related to a specific mood, create an "Emergency Emotional Pantry" with nutritious foods that will still satisfy your cravings without harming your body.

Knowledge is power to change! Choose to discover your emotional weaknesses, so you can effectively plan ahead.

**8. Six days shalt thou labor, but in the seventh day thou shalt rest.**
Everyone needs a break from time to time.

Dieting can be like babysitting a house full of kids—if you don't take a mental break it can make you crazy! Going 24/7 is expected of the ambitious in every aspect of life today, but I believe mental play time is critical to our dieting success.

> **FACT:** It is okay to take a "diet time out" if you need it!
> Choosing to take consistent small steps is much
> better than falling completely down the staircase.

This may seem shocking to you, but it's okay to take a break from this diet if you've reached your mental or physical limits. Why would a doctor write a diet book and then tell you its okay to not follow the diet strictly? Because diets that are too strict cause people to burn out instead of burning calories. They retreat defeated and beaten by completely dropping the diet.

"Rome wasn't built in a day"—and neither will your new and improved physique appear overnight. It takes substantial time and food to store fat and become fat, so it shouldn't be a surprise that it takes some time to deconstruct it as well.

Choosing to be consistent over time is more important than choosing to defeat yourself with too strict a regimen.

### 9. Honor thy family by succeeding together.

What good is success if those dearest to you don't also enjoy it?

Can you imagine looking and feeling great while the rest of your family is still sinking in the sticky, smelly fat swamp?

> **FACT:** You will feel like a superhero if you help your entire family become healthier.

Be a better mother, father, sister, brother, daughter, or son by practicing the Golden Rule—treat them the same way you would want to be treated. If you knew your mom was boarding a bus that was headed over a cliff, I think you would warn her and do everything you could to stop her from boarding that bus. Why then would you not warn her of the dangers of being overweight?

Leaving your family with a rich nutritional heritage is more important than leaving them monetary riches! Families cherish generational traditions and common ties. Heritage, after all, is something to be celebrated—from hair and eye color to endearing mannerisms and timeless stories. Recent studies, however, have found that there is one behavior that, when passed down, can be extremely detrimental to your health—poor eating habits and lifestyle.

Children with an obese parent are three times as likely to be obese when they reach adulthood, and children with two obese parents are ten times (1000 percent!) as likely. Why not pass down good habits to your children instead? You have the power through your actions and tongue to create a positive haven of health for your family in a raging sea of societal dietary sins.

You can choose today to become the nutritional champion that fights for your family's health and nutritional heritage. By helping others, you become stronger and more empowered.

Realize that you have the power to change your environment, the foods that surround you, and your family's health. Try an after dinner bonding walk with your spouse—where you talk, share the day, and unwind as you walk.

Let your kids and grandkids make critters out of fruit and veggies—using toothpicks to hold them together. Kids love making food sculptures, will cherish the memory, and enjoy eating them as much, or more, than home-made cookies.

As mom says, "This is real lovin'—with or without the oven."

## 10. Thou shalt not take thy diet strategy lightly.

Are you guilty of trying to cut corners with risky diet strategies—diet gimmicks that you know probably don't work and could even be dangerous or deadly to your health?

It's easy to believe miraculous claims because we *want* to believe they are true! We hear what we want to hear—that we can simply take a pill to quickly reverse years of dietary damage to our weight. Let me assure you that if such a pill existed, the world's largest pharmaceutical companies would have already sent a small army to seize it.

**FACT:** "Quid est veritas?" In case you don't speak Latin, that means "What is truth?" This is always the most important question you can ask about any diet.

The Truth: There are no shortcuts—no magic pills. Losing weight sensibly and safely requires realistic weight loss goals, reduced calorie intake, and adequate exercise as part of a clinically proven plan.

The good news is that I've done more than seven years of clinical research on the *Revival Slim and Beautiful Diet*, documenting amazing results that you can believe and trust.

Choose not to be duped into believing false claims that you can lose weight effortlessly—you are too smart to be fooled.

---

## DIET SCAMS LIST
### (ADAPTED FROM THE FDA)

There's an "I wanna be skinny tomorrow!" sucker born every minute. Don't let it be you.

- *Low-carb diets that encourage over-consumption of fatty foods.* The American Heart Association has stated that these diets can lead to premature heart disease.

- *Any diet, pill, capsule, juice, etc. that claims to help you lose a large amount of weight in a very short amount of time.* For example, a product that claims to help you lose 10 pounds over the weekend. This type of diet is very dangerous.

- *Diet patches, which are worn on the skin, have not been proven to be safe or effective.* The FDA has seized millions of these patches from manufacturers and promoters.

- *Fat blockers purport to physically absorb fat and mechanically interfere with the fat a person eats.* Anything that truly blocks fat absorption also blocks absorption of important vitamins, minerals, and other nutrients.

- *Carbohydrate blockers, sugar blockers, or starch blockers that promise to block or impede starch digestion.* Not only is the claim unproven, but users have complained of nausea, vomiting, diarrhea, and stomach pains.

- *Over-the-counter (OTC) diet pills.* A recent diet pill ingredient (phenyl-propanolamine or PPA) found in leading brand-name diet pills was removed from the market by the FDA due to increased risk of hemor-rhagic (bleeding) stroke. Nobody knows what the next disaster will be among OTC diet pills!

- *Magnet diet pills allegedly flush fat out of the body.* The FTC has brought legal action against marketers of these pills.

- *Bulk fillers that promise to swell in the stomach, thereby reducing hunger.* Some fillers can even prove harmful, causing obstructions in the intestines, stomach, or esophagus.

- *Electrical muscle stimulators have legitimate use in physical therapy treatment.* But the FDA has taken a number of them off the market because they were promoted for weight loss and body toning. When used incorrectly, muscle stimulators can be dangerous, causing elec-trical shocks and burns.

Choose not to be a sucker who believes nutty claims made by nuts. If it sounds too good to be true, it probably is! Check out the research, as well as who did the research, to make sure it was done at a reputable medical research facility.

You can get off the diet couch now! Try some stretching to get ready for a brisk walk. Our first session wasn't too painful was it?

Okay, if it was hurtful, remember it's a good hurt—a hurt that will help you get better, rather than stay stuck in a rut.

## BOTTOM LINE

I hope these commandments have given you a smarter mind to make your body permanently slimmer.

You need to check-in on this chapter often to help you get rid of ugly, gelatinous fat. Study these commandments until they are at your mental fingertips. When temptation threatens, form a mental fist and defend your health and life.

Do you hear what I'm saying? Stop sedating your true mind with false cupcakes, and start using your superhero psychological powers for good . . . the good of your permanent weight loss and better skin, hair, and nails!

And, just in case this chapter *has* been too brutally honest, I asked mom to give us a teaspoonful of sugar to help the psychological medicine go down.

### MOM'S BRIGHT BITE

I told Doc to take it easy on you, but I can see that my children listen less as they grow older. This will make you feel better in no time:

A very old couple was killed in an unfortunate accident. An angel was giving them a tour of heaven: "Here is your ocean-side mansion, over there are the tennis courts, swimming pool, and two golf courses. Your full-time massage therapists and gourmet chefs are available 24/7 by dialing 777. Your new Mercedes, BMW, and Ferrari are parked in the rear. Here are your credit cards with an unlimited spending amount. I recommend you visit our Rodeo Drive and Fifth Avenue. Our universe-class spa gives great facials and aromatherapy sessions."

"Heck, Roy," the old woman snarled as the angel flew off, "we could have been here fifteen years ago if you hadn't read about all that stupid soy protein, oat bran, wheat germ, and health food!"

—Anonymous

## CHAPTER 4

# Beauty and the Beanstalk: "I've Got Soy Under My Skin!"

*I'm tired of all this nonsense about beauty being only skin-deep.
That's deep enough. What do you want—an adorable pancreas?*
—JEAN KERR

> With Revival, my nails, hair, and skin look wonderful, and I feel like myself
> again.
>
> —V. IVANCIK, Results not typical.[†]

> I have been using Revival products daily. My skin is softer, my nails are
> stronger, my energy level is high, and people always comment on how well I
> look. It's great stuff!
>
> —N. ROSETTI, Results not typical.[†]

> Revival makes me feel better and my very dry skin is more moisturized.
>
> —A. FORD, Results not typical.[†]

Looking great isn't vanity—it's victory! Looking great makes us feel emotionally great, and that's vital for our longevity. So we should never even think twice that wanting to look better is somehow wrong.

---

[†]Results not typical, but included to motivate you. Individual results vary. You must follow the calorie-restricted diet plan, physical activity plan, and dietary supplement regimens presented in this book if you hope to achieve great weight loss, beauty, and health results. see *Introduction* and specific studies presented in this book for typical results. These statements have not been evaluated by the Food and Drug Administration. Revival is not intended to diagnose, treat, cure, or prevent any disease.

My recent research has documented that victory starts inside in our nutritional war against the unsightly appearance of fine lines, wrinkles, dull hair, and brittle nails. I'll lead the way as we learn about Revival's breakthrough nutritional makeover beauty results and "The Seven Deadly Skin Sins" to flee at all costs.

---

**FACT:** Even if you are constantly slathering yourself with the best quality creams, serums, shampoos, and polishes on the market, you are only doing fifty percent of what you could be doing to reduce the appearance of wrinkled, discolored skin; dull, unmanageable hair; and weak, brittle nails.

---

Topical applications are only 50 percent of the advanced weaponry available to use in our fight. To me that's an eye-opening-sit-up-straight-and-listen fact that can't be ignored.

Are you shocked to learn that eating the right foods and supplements can dramatically improve the appearance of your skin, hair and nails *from within*? "From within" is the remaining 50 percent of fighting our deteriorating appearance over time and may eventually prove to be the most important half! New studies continue to show that nourishing what we can't see below the surface has a dramatic impact on what we can see above the surface.

I was shocked to learn this, too. Working on appearance of skin from both ends is the *only* way for us to enjoy maximum beauty results.

Gorgeous skin, silky hair, and strong nails are like beautiful roses on a rose bush. Unless we nourish the roses and stems through the roots, the beautiful rose petals soon shrivel up with a sallow, pale color, and the stems begin to droop in floral disgrace, no matter how much topical water and nutrients we apply directly to the petals.

Want incredible beauty results? We have to go to the "invisible" root of the visible problems. I'll share my clinically proven "Exactly-What-To-Do" with you in this chapter.

## MOM'S BRIGHT BITE

A little girl was sitting on her grandmother's lap as she listened to a bedtime story. From time to time, the little girl would take her eyes off the book and reach up to touch her grandmother's wrinkled cheek. She was alternately stroking her own cheek, then her own again.

Finally she spoke up, "Grandma, did God make you?"

"Yes, sweetheart," she answered, "God made me a long time ago."

"Oh," she paused. "Grandma, did God make me, too?"

"Yes, He did, Honey," she said. "God made you just a little while ago."

Feeling of their respective faces again, she said, "God's getting better at it, isn't He?"

I love this hilarious, innocent, and honest child's-eye-view of aging. There's aging gracefully that is a normal part of the life cycle, and then there's premature, poor aging that we have a lot of power to prevent by choosing to enjoy the right beautifying foods!

## MOM'S "CLINK-CLINK" MADE ME START TO THINK . . .

A few months after mom started using the first Revival soy protein shake we formulated, she came to me and joyfully proclaimed, "I think my nails are getting stronger!" (And she simultaneously rolled her fingers several times against my desk so I could hear her fingernails clink-clink sharply one after the other against the wood.) I stopped for a moment to think before coming to my senses and bluntly quipped, "That's nice, Mom, but I'm trying to focus on something important right now." With a disappointed-at-my-disinterest look on her face, she turned around and walked briskly out of my office.

I didn't make much of her comment at the time, but a few weeks later I started noticing that she had a new glow radiating from her face with smoother-looking skin (dad described it as "rosy and beautiful"). Her skin color appeared warmer. Instead of looking "washed out," as so many people do when they age, mom started looking brighter and bouncier. She looked very healthy for the first time in a very long time. Dad and I could see the better health in her eyes.

By the end of the sixth month, it was clear from mom's better, silkier hair that something very positive had occurred (and was continuing to occur). But neither mom nor I had a clue as to why Revival would produce unexpected beauty benefits. I didn't have to ask if she was sure her skin, hair, and nails looked rejuvenated because Dad and I could easily see it for ourselves. *Was the soy getting under her skin?*

To be honest, I didn't have time to care much at the time. So what if mom had better-looking skin, hair, and nails? Her hot flashes were virtually gone, her waist was shrinking, she was sleeping very well, her Tasmanian Devils had been chased away, and she had more energy than I enjoyed! I had *serious* health research to work on that couldn't be bothered by silly cosmetic matters.

As you can gather by now, I'm a big believer in clinical trials to prove health claims. I was working on serious research for promotion of normal cholesterol health—you know, the really important *life-changing* stuff. I couldn't be bothered by possible trivial beauty benefits, no matter how much mom continued to rave about her skin, hair, and nails.

My ugly thinking soon took a turn for the better. Mom's new-looking skin, hair and nails weren't an isolated cosmetic anomaly. The beauty testimonies started coming in from Revival-LITES all over the country, compelling testimonies of life-changing improvements in appearance. Passionate praise for Revival's beauty benefits kept rolling in to our laboratory. I would read in amazement the testimonies late at night when I found time to take a short break from working on my "serious" research. Doing so began to deeply impact my beliefs about mom's silly beauty benefits. I learned something very important.

I learned that beauty isn't silly; it's emotionally sacred. Feeling great but not looking great is not great, it's awful. But, feeling great and looking great is amazing, it's life-changing. Pause for a moment and reread those last two sentences slowly—I want to make sure you understand what I'm saying before walking further.

**FACT:** Life tastes better when you feel more beautiful.

Do you understand what I'm saying? Mom describes the feeling well with a bright smile and sparkle in her eyes, "Beautiful skin, hair, and nails *taste* amazing."

Let's listen in to a few more testimonials to see just how "delicious" living a beautiful life can be when "gelatinous" is turned into "gorgeous."

*The most benefit I've had with Revival has been a general feeling of energy that I didn't have before, and also menopause discomforts have lessened. People tell me my skin looks so young. At sixty-two, I tell them it is Revival.*

—L. WELCH, Results not typical.[†]

*I have been enjoying Revival products for just over a year now, and I am thrilled with the taste and the results of improved health. I am forty-three years old raising a nine- and five-year-old. My hair has returned to its full body condition, as well as my skin (now dewy), and my nails are much stronger. The mood swings are stabilized as well as the cravings for sugar, chocolate, etc. I recommend your products to friends and family—and I am proud to do this knowing the integrity of your products. Keep up the great work you do in improving lives.*

—B. UTECH, Results not typical.[†]

*I am writing to tell you how happy I am since taking Revival. It has done wonders for me. My hair has improved, and I look and feel so much better and happier. I commend your efforts and wish you much success.*

—H. SINGER, Results not typical.[†]

*Two years ago, a friend of mine told me her doctor recommended Revival. Since I have begun taking it, my skin looks so much better. (I am sixty-seven years old.) It has regained moisture again. I can honestly say my appearance, health, and attitude is much better.*

—R. CARNEAL, Results not typical.[†]

*My fingernails are firm and hard—no splitting or peeling, for the first time in my life and better than when I was a teenager. And I've tried everything to grow nails. Revival has diminished, and at times eliminated, my hot flashes, so I sleep better at night.*

—P. FLORENCE, Results not typical.[†]

Do you think it's better to look good than to feel good? Many of us feel exactly this way, but why should we ever be content settling for just one or the other?

I don't know about you, but mom and I are having our cake and eating it too. Based on my medical research, you can have both physical health inside and physical beauty outside—a life you can love living.

The sweet taste of success is just down the hill. Are you still walking with me? Ready to run?

Do you know why I'm so excited that this diet will make you look better on the outside? Because you will experience a side-effect when you see a slimmer, sexier new you in the mirror—motivation. I'm confident that as you are brushing your softer, silkier hair; or painting your longer, stronger nails; or receiving compliments on your smoother-looking skin, you will feel motivated to continue making wise eating choices. And, those wise eating choices will make you more beautiful on the inside—

and that makes me very happy as a medical research doctor. It's *serious*.

What we see on the outside of our bodies as we age is also occurring on the inside of our bodies. Think about it: The deterioration we see in our wrinkled skin, dulling hair, and splitting nails is simply a "temperature gauge" for what is going on under our skin. Our brain, heart, blood vessels, lungs, digestive tract, liver, kidneys, reproductive organs, muscles, and bones are also becoming wrinkled with deterioration over time. Can you see it in your mind?

Can you feel it happening? Do you want to change it?

So, yes, we definitely do want an adorable pancreas—an *extremely* adorable pancreas and heart and arteries and brain and bones and . . . well, you get the picture. If our dietary changes are producing great visible results on the outside, we can assume that we are also supporting better health and looking "cuter" on the inside. Realizing this gave me a different appreciation for the often repeated statement, "I'm a beautiful person on the inside." Now when I hear someone say that, I automatically wonder, *Is she really more beautiful on the inside?*

---

### MOM'S BRIGHT BITE

Try this compliment out on your loved ones, "Wow! Your lungs are looking really cute lately." You will get some very puzzled looks, but it's a great way to start sharing what you are learning with those you love most.

**WARNING:** Not recommended for use on complete strangers!

---

Let me ask you several "critical care" questions:

- Are you delivering the right nutrients to your rose petals and stems via your roots?
- Do your petals look vibrant with color and plump with moisture?

- Are your stems arched gracefully?
- Are you starving your outward beauty without even realizing it?

What do you have under your skin?

## AND, BEHIND DOOR #1 WE HAVE . . .

We all know that our skin starts looking thin and saggy with age due to decreased collagen (which plumps the skin with volume) and elastin (which helps hold up the skin with elasticity). It's just an ugly fact of life that without intervention, we lose about 50 percent of our collagen by age fifty (yikes!).

Numerous factors other than aging accelerate this process, including declining estrogen levels during midlife. Decreased estrogen can lead to incredibly disturbing decreases in skin hydration (including the vaginal tissues) and collagen content; thinner, slower-growing hair; and, weaker, slower-growing nails. Excessive exposure to sunlight, poor dietary habits, stress, and cigarette smoking are also beauty killers.

### MOM'S BRIGHT BITE

*Fifty percent collagen loss?!!* It makes me want to shout Scooby Doo's famous line: "Rut-row!"

"Uh-oh" for sure if we choose to do nothing about it. I'm not going to get stuck in the midlife rut with poor-looking skin. I'm going to row to beauty safety by nourishing my skin, hair, and nails from within. Watch out aging! Beware of my new hard, strong nails . . . I will use them to defend my allure when needed.

Coco Chanel said, "Nature gives you the face you have at twenty. Life shapes the face you have at thirty. But at fifty you get the face you deserve." In addition to popularizing the little black dress, Coco is credited for starting our obsession with collagen-obliterating sun tanning (after she returned from a vacation brown and bronzed). Coco's quote is true, but the good news is that we don't have to fear the bad news, because we now have new skin-care research breakthroughs. Coco's last sentence should now read, "But at fifty you get the face you *choose*!" Even though what we do in our twenties and thirties will echo into midlife, we don't have to settle for less-than-gorgeous-looking skin any longer. We can *choose* magnificent over mediocre.

Will you choose Door #1 or Door #2? Let me give you a peek at what is behind each.

## Behind Door #1 we have, for your viewing pleasure:

Noticeably visible fine lines and wrinkles on the forehead.

Sleepy-looking eyelids.

Dark appearance of circles under the eyes.

The look of droopy, fallen cheeks.

Sad-looking smile lines of smile lines and bulldog-like jowls.

And everyone's favorite face accessory: looking like you have "turkey neck."

Yes, but wait . . . there's even more visible pleasure to excite you!

As skin dries out in midlife, a rapidly worsening appearance of wrinkles with blotchy discolorations and a fine mosaic of "crepe-paper" texture become visible.

Depletion of fat below the skin, which normally makes the face look plump, produces a hollowed skeleton look with decreased round appearance of the face.

I could go on and on describing our future faces without intervention but, frankly, I'm getting too depressed—doctors have emotions, too! Next door, please.

## Behind Door #2 . . .

After realizing how *emotionally sacred* better beauty is to Revival users, and seeing how it directly impacts overall well–being by making people better on the inside, too, my intellectual curiosity took over.

Just because something is said over and over thousands of times doesn't mean it is true. I knew a clinical trial had to be performed to see if the little bean had undocumented beauty secrets hidden inside. It was a research study I could passionately pursue, because I knew that scientifically proving that Revival helped people look great on the outside would help them stay healthier on the inside. It would be a win-win situation with everyone getting exactly what they want.

Did this miracle-in-a-pod also possess the power to nurture one's sacred emotions? Could a creamy protein shake or crispy snack bar reveal younger-looking skin?

The idea still sounded pretty far-fetched to me at the time (about equal to a UFO sighting). Intellectually, my "beauty from within" theory was a very long mental distance from my mainstream medical education. But as I heard more and more people tell Mom she looked ten years younger than her age, and as waiters or cashiers repeatedly asked if she was my wife, I became convinced Revival was up to something good looking under her skin—something really good.

Unanswered questions begging for answers ran through my mind. I would even wake up at night thinking about them. I already knew from studying published research that topically applied soy antioxidants and soy peptides (little pieces of soy protein) in creams can produce startling reductions in the appearance of fine lines, wrinkles, and skin discolorations, while at the same time brightening skin complexion, but could *eating* soy do the same?

Could the research showing that women in Asia don't readily show signs of wrinkling until about fifty years old actually be due in part to their soy consumption? Could their soy-rich diets contribute to their pearl-like skin appearance? Could Revival's nutritionally complete soy protein and powerful, naturally concentrated soy antioxidants fight the look of aging?

Mom and I couldn't wait for the clinical trial to start!

The exciting details from an independent, dermatologist-conducted Revival study follow, but I'll give you a quick summary in case you are as anxious as my mom and I were: the results were beautiful.

## CLINICALLY PROVEN NUTRITIONAL MAKEOVER

"Statistically significant" (i.e. real) improvements were seen in appearance of skin wrinkling, discoloration, flaking, and roughness with Revival consumption.

**Percent of Women Showing Improvement**

| | |
|---|---|
| Overall — 6 mo. | **93%** |
| Wrinkles — 6 mo. | **67%** |
| Discoloration — 6 mo. | **40%** |
| Flaking — 6 mo. | **73%** |
| Roughness — 6 mo. | **67%** |

**HAIR:** Statistically significant improvements were seen in appearance of hair dullness, scalp flaking, manageability, and hair roughness with Revival consumption.

**Percent of Women Showing Improvement**

| | |
|---|---|
| Overall — 6 mo. | **53%** |
| Dullness — 6 mo. | **67%** |
| Scalp Flaking — 6 mo. | **67%** |
| Manageability — 6 mo. | **47%** |
| Roughness — 6 mo. | **67%** |

**NAILS:** Statistically significant improvements were seen in splitting, flaking, ridging, and nail roughness with Revival consumption.

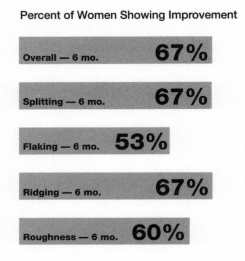

**Percent of Women Showing Improvement**

| | |
|---|---|
| Overall — 6 mo. | **67%** |
| Splitting — 6 mo. | **67%** |
| Flaking — 6 mo. | **53%** |
| Ridging — 6 mo. | **67%** |
| Roughness — 6 mo. | **60%** |

I had the answers to the questions running through my mind: yes, yes, yes, and yes!

The study results verified Revival's sexiest protein on the planet status (along with the clinically proven weight loss benefits). Not only were these beautiful results reported by the study participants (i.e., they could see the changes in their mirror for themselves), but more importantly, the improvements were documented by the independent dermatologist conducting the study.

Just so you realize the importance of this, let me explain further. Many cosmetic studies only document the opinion of a study's participants, for example, "In this study, 90 percent of women reported they saw better skin." However, in the Revival study the improvements were also documented by the dermatologist who concluded, "Improvements in appearance of skin, hair, and nails were evident after six months of Revival consumption, with some benefits being noted as early as three months." The results were clearly evident, visible, and real ("statistically significant").

## "ENOUGH SCIENCE! TELL ME EXACTLY-WHAT-TO-DO, NOW!"

Sounds like you are ready for sexier-looking skin, silkier hair, and stronger nails!

The women in the study, fifty to sixty-five years of age, with mild to moderate sun-damaged skin simply consumed one delicious naturally concentrated Revival soy serving, containing 20 grams of soy protein and 160 milligrams of soy antioxidants, per day.

So you simply need to enjoy one naturally concentrated Revival soy bar or shake supplement daily for beauty benefits—that's it!

It's easy to include one naturally concentrated bar or shake supplement as part of your daily eating pattern (as part of the milk-protein-based diet or soy-protein-based diet). And even if you aren't trying to lose weight on the diet, you can still enjoy improving the appearance of your skin, hair, and nails just by supplementing your diet with the bars and shakes.

---

**FACT:** It's easy to put the power of the sexiest protein on the planet to work for you.

---

The 20 grams of high-quality soy protein supplies our skin, hair, and nails with the basic building blocks (amino acids) needed to support a firm foundation. Milk protein also supplies these high-quality building blocks, so it may be possible to experience better-looking skin, hair, and nails with Revival milk-protein-based products. We are working on clinically testing them for beauty benefits. Milk protein, like soy protein, contains unique peptides that may support healthy connective tissue.

Soy has a lot of added antioxidant goodness for connective tissue support that isn't found in other protein sources. Soy antioxidants (isoflavones) may support our skin, hair, and nails by neutralizing unhealthy free radicals (a known cause of aging) generated by sun exposure, poor diet, and environmental pollution. Since topically applied soy antioxidants (and topically applied soy peptides) already have well documented beauty benefits, it isn't surprising that they can work from the inside too.

Unhealthy free radicals are like bulls in a China shop! Unless they are stopped they will shatter our health to pieces—including our connective tissue health—causing visible signs of aging. Fortunately, just one naturally concentrated Revival bar or shake supplement contains the same amount of soy antioxidants found in 6 cups of a typical soymilk. That's a powerful, neutralizing punch for the bulls!

"Naturally concentrated" is a reason to seriously celebrate, because it allows us to enjoy the full benefits of soy antioxidants easily in just one serving (not to mention the taste immersion). Revival is the only brand to contain this clinically proven form of naturally concentrated soy, because patents around the world protect it, even in China where soy originated thousands of years ago.

## MOM'S BRIGHT BITE

As the lady sat before her vanity mirror and gingerly applied her makeup, her husband entered the room. He stood in amazement as she added one thing after another to be beautiful. First her cheeks, then her eyes, then her lips. It all seemed to be taking form when she leaned toward the mirror, peered into it intently, and then lamented about how old she was looking. He hastily replied, "Well Darling, just sand it down and start over!"

Somebody probably earned a few days in the doghouse for that comment. Revival products are helping me continually "sand it down" from the inside out for a better-looking foundation.

Can we get the same benefits from a soy pill? Not likely because the soybean is a grand symphony of many different and good molecules, beyond just protein and antioxidants. Unless we have all of the instruments playing their beautiful roles in sweet unison, it just doesn't "sound" as good to your health. Your skin, hair, nails, and body needs both the protein and the antioxidants together.

If you want to get a head start on sexier-looking skin, hair, and nails, contact my friendly nutrition staff for expert nutritional makeover advice at **1-800-REVIVAL** (1-800-738-4825), **www.RevivalDiet.com**, or **Nutrition@RevivalDiet.com**.

## "DOC, I WANT TO LOOK TEN YEARS YOUNGER"

Let's say you came into my laboratory today and said, "Doc, I want to get serious about improving the health and appearance of my skin, hair and nails. How can you help me?"

I'd get out a pad, write the following list, hand it to you and ask you to come see me in three months:

### Flee the Seven Deadly Skin Sins

1. *Make a final decision today: "I am going to work daily to improve my skin, hair and nails."* Choosing to do little (or nothing) for your skin is the greatest deadly skin sin. Inaction will always kill your lustrous looks. Freezing in your tracks won't freeze time or gravity. You must take immediate action, and the earlier in life the better. By the time the captain of the Titanic saw the tip of the iceberg, it was too late to turn—the unseen danger below the surface fatally ripped the ship.

Choose to start taking care of your skin *today,* including use of a skincare regimen that you stay on for a minimum of three months. Frequent switching between brands does not give your skin enough time to respond properly.

## MOM'S BRIGHT BITE

Powder and paint? We girls have a real challenge with all this makeup . . . decisions, decisions, decisions! There is even makeup specifically advertised for women in their 20s, 30s, and 40s, but it mostly stops there. I tried the one for the 30s thinking it would do something for me, but guess what? All it did was make my puppy Yorkie growl at me! Must have been the iridescent green eye shadow I was playing around with for kicks. My dad used to say to me as a teenager, "Powder and paint makes people think you is what you ain't." I guess it can make your dog think you are someone else, too!

It is a real blessing that Revival helps me have smoother-looking skin, so I don't have to rely 100 percent on powder and paint to look great (but it is fun to try new colors from time to time). Consistently staying on Revival can help give you a natural "growl-free" glow, too.

*2. Supplement your way to suppleness: Perfect and protect younger-looking skin, hair, and nails!* Failure to use new clinically proven beauty supplement technology, including naturally concentrated Revival bars and shakes, is the second deadliest skin sin.

Why? New beauty-research breakthroughs, including Revival's research, prove that you can perfect and protect the appearance of your "rose petals and stems" from within. I'm not sure why anyone would refuse to benefit from this new nutritional makeover technology unless they have a Beauty IQ that needs a serious makeover!

Why not simply use whole foods? We've all heard other doctors talking about looking better by eating salmon, dairy foods, fruits, and veggies. While regular whole foods may help a little bit, they are too weak to produce a fast, dramatic visible change that you can clearly see. It's simply impossible to get enough skin-beneficial nutrients for significant changes to rapidly appear from whole foods. Eating more salmon, calcium-rich foods, and antioxidant-rich fruits and vegetables is a great first step, but don't expect doing that alone to put a *big* smile on your face when looking in the mirror without makeup on. A piece of salmon isn't as strong as concentrated fish oil. Soymilk isn't as strong as naturally concentrated Revival (which contains 600 percent more soy antioxidants than a typical soymilk). Tomatoes aren't as strong as concentrated lycopene extracts. Even calcium, very abundant in dairy foods, needs to be supplemented daily by most women. The best strategy is to *combine* beauty whole foods like salmon and antioxidant-rich fruits with concentrated beauty dietary supplements.

**FACT:** The beauty of using concentrated dietary supplements is that you can easily get enough of the "good stuff" that's simply impractical with whole foods. Who can eat a big bushel of berries every day?

The right concentrated ingredients can produce significant visible appearance changes. Concentration can make life better with noticeable changes in the look of your skin, hair, and nails.

## MY TWENTY BEST PERFECT-AND-PROTECT BEAUTY PEARLS!

Ready to start reaping the supple rewards of concentrated dietary supplementation?

I want to share with you my hand-picked list of what I call "My Twenty Best Perfect-and-Protect Beauty Pearls"—dietary supplement ingredients that have been clinically tested in human studies or laboratory studies. I hope you realize by now that I only recommend what is clinically tested!

Unfortunately, you can turn on almost any home-shopping channel, or pick up any book, or walk into any health food store or pharmacy, to find many "experts" with products making beauty claims based on sheer speculation. Follow the advice my mom gave to me growing up: "Don't take any wooden nickels." Insist on having proof of effectiveness.

If you are like my mom (i.e., too busy with life, kids, grandkids and a new puppy to take time to earn a Ph.D. in science), you just want the added sexy-strength benefits of the right dietary supplements. You don't want to have to figure out exactly which twenty separate products or brands to purchase at your local store (not to mention the high cost of so many separate bottles and wasted packaging materials). And you don't have the time or patience to open twenty or more different bottles every morning and night—someone pass the headache medicine, please!

I understand. Life is too short for you to have to earn a science degree just because you want to maximize your benefits from beauty supplements so I've formulated the perfect total-body beauty supplement with right ingredients. I've named the supplement "Gorgeous Roses" because it nourishes the appearance of your skin, hair, nails, and other body tissues tp help your outer beauty flourish like roses in full glorious bloom—while also supporting your full inner beauty health. All of the beauty goodness is power-packed into several small pills, so you don't agonize over opening twenty or more bottles per day (no one can stay faithful to such torment long-term). The formula also contains all the basic vitamins, minerals, and powerful antioxidants you need to support healthier weight loss and to maintain better health in every major organ in your body, so it is a real one-two-three beauty punch.

I like to think about all the right concentrated beauty ingredients diffused throughout my entire body, nourishing my skin, hair, nails, and every other cell, all working overtime to make me glow—inside and out. I don't like the thought of not having them perfecting, protecting, and promoting better health around the clock, so I choose to use the formula daily. It's a very simple choice. Let's discuss the ingredients that ignite beauty!

## My Twenty Best Perfect-and-Protect Beauty Pearls—for Kissable Benefits!

Let's take a look at your new "string of pearls." It's my gift to you to celebrate your new marriage to happier-looking skin, hair, and nails.

In addition to at least one Revival naturally concentrated soy bar or shake per day, embrace these recommendations for maximum kissable and huggable benefits:

1. **Olive-leaf extract.** concentrates the natural-beauty goodness found in olives. Addition of olive-leaf extract to the diet has been shown to promote antioxidant health and improve appearance of aging. *A little taste of Italy never sounded so beautiful.*

2. **Kiwi-seed extract.** Who knew a fruit also called the "Chinese gooseberry" would contain your Presidential-Suite tickets to the Stunning-Skin Ballet? Studies have shown that kiwi-seed extract improves radiance, reduces appearance of fine lines and dark circles, and improves skin moisture. *There must be some beautiful geese in China!*

3. **Shark cartilage** is a rich source of collagen and other molecules to support better-looking skin with increased hydration. *"Finding Nemo" is nice for your skin!*

4. **Muscadine grape powder (skin and seed).** Muscadines are a large grape variety found primarily "down South" in the United States. Muscadines are big on taste and huge on antioxidant content, with up to ten times the antioxidant power of blueberries and

cranberries. *Muscadine antioxidants can help your skin take a lickin' and keep on tickin.'*

5. **Milk-protein peptides.** It shouldn't be a surprise that little pieces of milk protein give you soft, smooth-looking "milky skin" by possessing some excellent beauty-promoting benefits. Milk-protein peptides may enhance your skin's emergency antioxidant system against environmental aggressions, thus helping to take a bite out of the visible signs of aging. *Pep up your skin with milk peptides from within!*

6. **Rosemary extract** will help keep your vibrant rose petals looking rosy by supporting cell membrane health. But don't reach for the spice rack, only a highly concentrated extract will do. *Marry into better skin with rosemary!*

7. **Cocoa extract.** Somebody please scream "yes" for chocolate! But don't pack on the pounds by trying to eat enough chocolate to look like a cherub. *A cocoa-rich Revival shake makes the perfect date, but reach for antioxidant-rich cocoa extract for concentrated skin delirium.*

8. **Astaxanthin** is a potent natural antioxidant found in Hawaiian-grown blue-green algae. So catch the wave with stronger-than-vitamin-E astaxanthin, proven to reduce appearance of skin discolorations and increase antioxidant health. *Hawaii-Five-Oh!-My-Skin-Looks-So-Good!*

9. **Tocotrienols,** a special type of vitamin E superhero, team with astaxanthin to reduce appearance of fine wrinkles and discolorations while smoothing and moisturizing the skin. *Go loco for Toco!*

10. **Green-tea extract.** The right highly concentrated green-tea extract, rich in tissue-supporting ECGC, makes it easy for you to enjoy the same beauty benefits as if you were sipping 4 to 8 cups of green tea per day. Better-looking skin can be a cup of tea with the right dietary ingredients that support normal DNA health. *Prevent your skin from needing an EKG by getting enough ECGC.*

11. **Lycopene.** Throw tomatoes at a dull appearance with the red plant

antioxidant lycopene. Instead of a tomato purée facial, snap up a highly concentrated lycopene extract. *Say "Bon Appétit!" to a rosier glow as you put some pink back into your pucker with lycopene.*

12. **Beta-carotene** is the orange pigment that gives carrots their warm glow. It's a building block for collagen-coddling retinol (vitamin A). Studies show beta-carotene has great-looking antioxidant benefits for your skin. *Make sure your roses bloom with beta-carotene's bona-fide antioxidant benefits!*

13. **Lutein.** Studies show you can put the power of Popeye the Sailor to work for your skin with increased moisture and stronger antioxidant health. Found naturally in spinach, lutein's eye-health support may also help you enjoy normal vision. *Sail away to a better-looking destination with lutein!*

14. **Biotin.** Build better bionic nails and healthier hair with biotin. Reach for 2.5 milligrams per day for maximum benefits. *Be hard on poor-looking nails and hair with biotin!*

15. **Borage oil.** Twice as strong as evening primrose oil, borage oil is naturally rich in the essential Omega-6 fatty acid ("essential" because our bodies can't manufacture it). *Look Omega-Sexier with Omega-Six from borage oil.*

16. **Alpha Lipoic Acid.** Able to see through walls and leap over tall buildings in a single bound, Alpha Lipoic Acid has been called the "super universal antioxidant." It works both inside and outside of cells to stop beauty crimes before they happen. *Support more innocent-looking skin faster than a speeding bullet with Alpha Lipoic Acid.*

17. **Enteric-coated fish oil.** Fish oil is swimming with Omega-3 essential fatty acids for total body health and beauty. Don't feel like stuffing yourself daily with a small school of salmon or sardines? I didn't think so, so I'll let you off the hook. *Enjoy enteric-coated fish-oil concentrate for all the benefits without the fishy aftertaste.*

18. **Flax-seed oil** complements fish oil as the perfect plant-based source of Omega-3 for the look of flourishing skin, hair, and nails. *Support sexier-looking skin in a flash with flax!*

19. **Coenzyme Q10.** Although Coenzyme Q10 has a funny-sounding name, its role in supporting energy production for every cell of your body, including our heart and skin, is no joke. "CoQ10," as his friends call him, may also support healthier cell membranes for healthier-appearing skin. *Enjoy CoQ10 to help you look like a "10"!*

20. **Calcium.** Yell "Calcium, take me away!" every day, because calcium is the firm foundation of normal bone health. Being bent over with bad bones and a camel hump isn't exactly beautiful, so make sure you are getting enough (the adequate daily intake of calcium for teens and adults ranges from 1000 to 1300 milligrams per day). *Stand up and shout if you have calcium deep down in you!*

    And while we are talking about bones, make sure you are facing the facts about facial aging. A recent study by the American Society of Plastic Surgeons found that shrinking facial bones is a significant contributor to facial aging. Skin elasticity diminishes with age, but your facial bones also change in shape, many times, dissolving and shrinking. These bone shifts often leave empty spaces in the face and accentuate drooping skin and wrinkles. Women experience a significant decrease in facial bone loss at an earlier age, meaning that the  sinking signs of aging strike women before they do men. So, make no bones about it, from the top of your head to the tip of your toes, calcium is vital for your total body beauty. *Calcium does a body good!*

## Bottom Line on Beauty Pearls

Studies suggest you can enjoy a significant improvement in your appearance by faithfully employing the right concentrated beauty ingredients, including naturally concentrated Revival bars and shakes, to help wash your worn looks away. Putting some cheer and bounce back into your skin, hair, and nails maximizes your kissable and huggable benefits. Your noticeable glow will soon warm every room graced by your presence.

In addition to my twenty best beauty pearls, it's also important to benefit from the tried-and-true skin-healthy vitamins and minerals (like vitamin C, which is vital for collagen metabolism, and zinc, which is critical to support proper function of your skin's most powerful detoxifying enzymes). My "Gorgeous Roses" formula contains the exact ones you need to nourish all of your body's tissues for better health support, including your skin, hair, nails, brain, eyes, heart, cardiovascular system, lungs, digestive tract, liver, kidneys, muscle, bones, and of course, your adorable pancreas—everything inside and outside. I update the formula regularly to add in new beauty-research technologies based on clinical research, so you don't have to do anything but "sit there and look pretty!"

Choose to lose your dull appearance by putting the power of more than twenty clinically tested ingredients to work on your roses. People are going to say your rose petals look fabulous and your stems look firm. You can contact my nutrition staff for more information on the picture-perfect beauty solution by calling **1-800-REVIVAL** (1-800-738-4825), or by logging on to **www.RevivalDiet.com**, or **Nutrition@RevivalDiet.com**.

To finish polishing off your new pearl-like appearance, drink as much ice-cold water or other calorie-free fluids as you can (unsweetened tea—green or black—adds extra antioxidants to your efforts). Not only will it help you burn calories and keep joints better cushioned, but constant hydration will also help your skin stay supple and sexy (while removing toxins from your body). Mom and I both reach for ultra-pure bottled water instead of spring water because it is cleaner and healthier, without toxins or inorganic matter that can potentially tear down the look of our skin, hair, and nails. The near future of fluids is looking great—I'm currently working on a new beauty water with liposomes containing beauty vitamins, minerals, and antioxidants.

Let's end this skin sin on a sweet note by remembering that lower blood-sugar levels may help keep your skin looking more succulent. Reach for low-glycemic foods that don't cause rapid rises in blood sugar. Why? Abnormal blood-sugar levels may accelerate the visible signs of aging by accelerating an aging process that "clots" your collagen and elastin fibers. Clotted collagen and elastin hinders the normal cycle of renewal, and that's a very bad situation for a budding diva's skin appearance.

3. *Avoid smoking and second-hand smoke at all costs.* Smoke is, without a doubt, "of the devil" when it comes to skin health. If you are still smoking, or regularly breathing in the four thousand chemicals in smoke second-hand, you "need to have your head examined," as my granddad used to say with a grin. Twin observation studies show that smoking will make you look like the Wicked Witch of the West faster than Toto can scarf down a Milk-Bone doggie treat.

So before you find yourself not in beautiful Kansas any longer, choose to avoid smoke at all costs. Red slippers never look good on a wrinkled witch anyway!

4. *Avoid the devil's darts: Use sunscreen religiously.* The sun's rays are the Devil's Darts that slay your skin's appearance.

Sounds like a cheap horror film preview to me! Prevent "sun screams" with generous use of sunscreens. You will reap what you sow when it comes to sun exposure. Even though new skin-care technologies (e.g., soy peptides) can help reverse the visible signs of prior sun damage, an ounce of prevention applied to your face daily in the form of a moisturizing sunscreen will keep your beauty from getting pounded. And the extra moisture will help seal in your skin's goodness.

**FACT:** UVA and UVB rays literally cause your cell membrane lipids to become rancid (i.e., rot); fatally damage your collagen and elastin genes by making new collagen and elastin synthesis impossible; activate millions of tiny collagen-snipping scissors that cut your collagen into millions of tiny pieces; quickly deplete your skin's natural antioxidant defenses; and start an inflammation cycle that can smolder on and on.

Reach for at least SPF 20 to stay looking as close to twenty as possible. Make sure it blocks both UVA and UVB darts. Many people make the mistake of only applying in the summer or on sunny days, but you should apply it every day (even if it is hazy or cloudy). Stay in the routine—you wouldn't skip a day brushing your teeth would you? (If you would, then you need a lot more help than this book offers!)

Reapply your sunscreen every few hours and make sure even the tiny places are covered. Don't forget the back of your neck, the back of your hands, and the tops of your ears, one place where skin cancer loves to make a debut performance; you definitely don't want to join the skin cancer party that more than 62,000 Americans attend each year. Use sun-protecting lipstick or lip balm.

Women are most susceptible to dart damage the week before a period, so wear extra sunscreen and avoid harsh face treatments during that time.

**FACT:** Winning the "Best Tan Award"
is not an honor—it's health heresy!

Dodge the darts by avoiding direct sun exposure between 10 a.m. to 4 p.m. (peak hours). If you are still going to a tanning bed or basking for long hours in the hot sun, you obviously weren't disciplined enough as a child! It makes me want to ask you, "What would you do with a brain if you had one?" I'm trying to say it in the nicest way possible: STOP!!! Use self-tanners as your personal save-my-skin campaign alternative.

Keeping every inch of your body's skin moisturized, not the just your decorative parts, is important for your face. How? Think of a water balloon with lots of tiny water streams coming out of lots of tiny holes. It doesn't matter if you fix half the tiny leaks because the balloon will still deflate and become droopy. Using a super moisturizer *only* on your face and not the rest of the body is simply not enough fingers to keep your delicious, skin dam from bursting. Even if your skin doesn't feel dry, a moisturizer can still seal in more hydration for better long-term results. Plus, applying a full-body moisturizer at least once per day—morning *and* night would be better—all the way down to the tips of your toes is a great way to get your daily stretching in. With a little practice and weight loss, you might even be able to reach all of your back, too!

## MOM'S BRIGHT BITE

I read that if mice eat soy they enjoy healthier-looking skin even after sun exposure. It got me to thinking, "How in the world do they study mice and sun exposure anyway?" I can just imagine all of them relaxing on the beach with their tiny black sunglasses, enjoying cheese or digging holes in the sand. I guess even mice should always wear sunscreen. A bronzed, wrinkled Mickey and Minnie wouldn't be a pretty sight!

Wear a hat, sunglasses (with 100 percent UV absorption) and clothes made of tightly-woven fabric if you do have to be in the sun to protect your hair, eyes, and body. Look for new hats and clothes with built-in sun protection.

Make sure your healthcare provider gives your skin a thorough exam at least once yearly to detect any suspicious changes. Early detection can save your life, so you play a critical role in monitoring your skin's integrity. Immediately have your healthcare provider examine any change you see on your skin, particularly if the size or color of a mole or other darkly pigmented spot changes, or if a spot starts oozing, bleeding, hurting, or itching.

Choose to block the Devil's darts by putting on the whole armor of sunscreen!

*5. Get your hand out of your mom's cookie jar: Apply topical soy peptides.* Get your hand out of your mother's skin-care-product cookie jar! Just because "Mom used it" doesn't means its still as good as it used to be. Newer, better technologies exist. In fact, many large cosmetic companies chose cheap ingredients over the latest age-defying technologies. In my opinion they don't truly want to help you. Why would the same cosmetic company have eight different nighttime repair creams? Because they know you will eventually purchase all eight in desperation. So don't become a victim of the great cosmetic cover-up. Why would you trust your skin's serious future to any cosmetic company that also makes sparkly lipstick? So try the latest new technologies. Here is one of my favorites:

*Topically applied soy peptides* have been shown to reduce the appearance of fine lines and wrinkles, reduce skin discolorations, and brighten skin complexion. With so many soy peptides available now it can be confusing, so I've researched and selected the cream of the crop. I've put the best of the best clinically proven soy peptides, along with more than ten other clinically tested next-generation ingredients, into a luxurious topical cream. It can be used alone or in combination with your existing skin care regimen. It's modernized frequently (just like the rest of our formulas are updated frequently).

Combined with Revival's naturally concentrated bars, shakes, and perfect-and-protect "Gorgeous Roses" dietary supplement, the soy peptide topical cream is a powerful way to work on reducing the visible signs of aging from both ends. Think of soy peptides as your beauty butler—willing and able to serve up delicious, gourmet glamour for your skin on command.

Choose to be a smart cookie by smoothing your skin's appearance with the latest smart technologies. You can contact my Nutrition Staff or visit **www.RevivalDiet.com** for more information on these and other new beauty boosting technologies that I'm researching and developing.

6. *Say goodbye to your poor lifestyle.* A poor lifestyle, which makes your skin look poor, is our next deadly skin sin. Gluttonous stuffing from the all-you-can-eat buffet line of uncontrolled stress, lack of sleep, and no exercise quickly blows up your beauty dreams.

Take immediate, drastic corrective action before you end up in the emergency room with an ugly case of skin, hair, and nail mediocrity. Just do whatever it takes to change! Remember a brisk walk can lower your stress, improve your mood, and help bring out a rosy glow in your skin and a sparkle in your eyes.

7. *Don't over treat your skin.* Cleanliness *is* next to godliness in skin care, but too much of a good thing is bad. Excessive treatment of your skin with harsh cleansers and scrubs turn fabulous into foul. Think less is more if you are experiencing irritation or breakouts.

### MOM'S BRIGHT BITE

Facial features are what they are . . . unless you hire a good plastic surgeon to change them! But improving what we have without surgery is always the best path.

Choose facial cleansers, soaps, and shampoos that do *not* contain sodium laureth sulfate and sodium dodecyl sulfate (or anything that sounds similar).

These chemicals are known to activate more than fifty inflammatory genes in your skin. Beware of scrubs that contain sharp-edged fruit seeds, which can cause microscopic punctures (that bacteria adore) in your delicate skin if used too vigorously.

I'm often asked if plastic surgery, chemical peels, microdermabrasion, laser surgery, intense pulsed-light therapy and other skin resurfacing treatments are too much ,or are they worthwhile. If you have significant damage from your past, a small "touch up" may be worth the risks. In fact, resurfacing treatments can remove precancerous cells. But moderation is always the best policy. Even if you choose strong medical treatments, you still need to continue eating the right concentrated beauty ingredients and using the latest beauty technologies (like soy peptides) to prevent continued deterioration in your appearance. Having a laser resurfacing treatment doesn't stop your skin from resuming its natural degradation the moment you walk out of the doctor's office.

Choose to help your skin be all it can be by knowing when enough is enough.

## BOTTOM LINE: REPENT AND YOUR SKIN SHALL BE SAVED!

If learning about new sin-free beauty research is "yummy" to you, stay up to date with my latest research and recommendations at **www.RevivalDiet.com**.

Don't forget the power of perception. How you apply your makeup, how you style your hair, and what clothes you wear all have a tremendous impact on how others (and yourself) perceive your beauty. Although we all want our skin, hair, and nails to look "stuck in time," having the rest of our appearance (makeup, haircut, and clothes) look "stuck in time" is not a pretty picture.

Get a makeover (free at the cosmetic counter of your choice). Add some color to your life (if your dog barks at you it probably isn't the right color or shade). Tell your stylist to change it up a bit. Go on a shopping spree for that little red dress. *Conquer!*

When you act as beautifully, regally, and nobly as you were created to be, others will perceive you to be more beautiful, and they may even change themselves for the better, too, as they wonder, *What does she have inside that makes her glow?*

Choose to be an angelic light by saying no to the darkness of deterioration. You know exactly what to do—choose Door #2. And since my mom taught me to be a Southern gentleman, let me open the door for you. . . .

## MOM'S BRIGHT BITE

Has Mona Lisa lost her smile?

Have you noticed that the scales of outward beauty change with the age, society, and culture we live in? By today's standards, most of us would have to admit that Mona Lisa isn't exactly a fox. Have you noticed she has no eyebrows or eyelashes? Had we lived in Mona Lisa's time, we would have felt compelled to pull out all of our eyelashes and eyebrows because it was considered unsightly for "genteel ladies" . . . ouch! The worst thing I ever personally did in the name of beauty was to iron my hair after bleaching it when I was sixteen.

The fact is that beauty is and always will be in the eye of the beholder. We like long eyelashes and perfectly trimmed eyebrows in this day and age. We think smooth skin, shiny hair, and long nails are beautiful. We see being slim as sexy. It could all change soon. So instead of debating about the changing beauty of Mona Lisa's smile, we should focus on what we know is true and will never change: eating the right foods makes us beautiful on the inside—past, present, and future. That's a fact that should make all of us smile.

## CHAPTER 5

# The Fifteen Physical Laws
# of Accelerated Weight Loss

The *Revival Slim & Beautiful Diet* produces amazing results when used alone, but you can seal the victory in the nutritional war by uniting your new superhero psychological powers you've gained from my "Ten Psychological Commandments of Permanent Weight Loss" with my "Fifteen Physical Laws of Accelerated Weight Loss."

Doing so will make you a formidable Superwoman or Superman in your fight against the fat felons!

Fatman and Boy Blubber? No. The Incredible Hunk and Purrr-woman, yes!

## 1. GOT A "DIET BUDDY"? START A FRIENDLY
## WEIGHT LOSS COMPETITION WITH HIM OR HER!

A friendly diet competition can be an extremely powerful motivator with a spouse, friend, or co-worker. A single parrot can learn about fifty words through regular training, but two parrots competing for food can learn more than two thousand words each! But a little healthy competition isn't just for the birds—use a Diet Buddy to double your weight loss pleasure as you both lose the double bubbles.

Start competing to see who can lose the most pounds. A "Weekly Weigh-In" with your Diet Buddy by phone or e-mail keeps the competition going, and keeps you both accountable to maximize results. During the weigh-in, share and celebrate your successes (was it a saint week or sinner week?), and discuss how to overcome your weaknesses. Specifically discuss how faithful each of you are being to your daily eating patterns and how you can tighten up any shortcomings.

Act as a lifeline for each other in temptation emergencies! A quick phone call to your Diet Buddy can help you make a win decision when you're crumbling under pressure.

You can create a free online Diet Buddy Group at **www.RevivalDiet.com/Resources** that allows you and your Diet Buddy (or Diet Buddies) to track your nutritional makeover improvements together (and easily hold each other accountable).

Choose your Diet Buddy wisely—find someone you know will motivate you and vice-versa as a team.

---

## MOM'S BRIGHT BITE

Who not to choose when looking for your Diet Buddy:

Renee and Sue were best of friends and tried to do everything together. Renee announced that she was going to start a diet to lose some pounds.

"Good," Sue exclaimed. "I'm ready to start a diet, too. We can be dieting buddies and help each other out."

"Perfect," replied Renee. "And when I feel the urge to drive out and get a burger and fries, I'll call you first."

"Great," Sue shouted. "I'll ride with you to get it!!!"

Don't have an overweight friend to be your Diet Buddy? Then grab a family member or close friend. They will volunteer if they care about your health.

You can also find a Diet Buddy (or Diet Buddy group to join) at our website.

Share the love and become a shrink by starting and leading a Revival Diet Small Group in your local area with a weekly structured teaching and group accountability meeting. See exactly how to do it in the *Resources to Rule Your World* section of this book (we supply all of the small group teaching materials for free at **wwwRevivalDiet.com/Resources**). You will become stronger by leading others. You can literally help change and save lives!

## 2. GET RID OF YOUR FAT FRIENDS AND FAMILY.

WOW! Why? Because fat is infectious—"birds of a feather flock together."

Peer pressure is a very powerful and controlling influence on unhealthy eating choices. Ever tried to order a healthy salad or meal when everyone else is ordering bacon cheeseburgers with French fries and milkshakes? Even if you do order healthy food, it isn't long before you are picking at their plates. Sometimes the toughest part of a diet isn't watching what you eat— it's watching all the food that other people eat!

> **FACT:** Your fat friends and family may be making you ugly and gelatinous with their negative eating influences.

Don't allow them to sabotage your health any longer. Does this sound too harsh? Well, then let me ask you a question: Are you doing the same to them by being a negative dietary influence? Maybe they should get rid of *you*.

Friends don't let friends die fat. I hope you understand my point.

Here's the happy alternative (before I get too many angry letters!): Instead of getting rid of your fat friends and family, help them lose weight with you.

Technically, you are still partially getting rid of them, but only the unhealthy ugly parts—the fat part.

Be a leader and tell your friends and family to "shape up or ship out!"

---

**FACT:** Women fulfill critical roles in our society's businesses, charitable groups, churches, and families. You may be the *only* help your family will ever get, so fight fiercely as the health gatekeeper for your entire family.

---

If they have simply stopped trying, and simply don't care any longer, it's up to you—the superhero—to resuscitate their self-esteem and motivation. Remember that one bad apple can ruin the whole bunch if something isn't done to repair the bad apple.

---

### MOM'S BRIGHT BITE

Women should play a special health gatekeeper role in the family. I have become the food police for my home to help out my husband (guys get middle-age spread, too!). I can hear every cabinet door open and can even track his moves by the trail of crumbs. It reminds me of the story about another husband and wife investigation:

**WIFE TO HER FAT HUSBAND:** Last night there were two pieces of cake in the refrigerator and now there is only one. How do you explain that?
**HUSBAND:** I guess it was so dark that I didn't see the other piece.

---

If your spouse is dragging you down to the grave, tell him or her it is high time for a dietary divorce. The two of you are going to divorce yourselves from the negative eating influences invading your home. Give negativity a Kung Fu kick out of your house.

## 3. GO ON A SHOPPING SPREE FOR NEW DISHES.

Don't you just love a doctor that tells you to go shopping? First new walking shoes and outfits and now dishes! Why? Studies show that dish color and dish size can drastically impact your hunger levels and how much food you eat.

You've heard the phrase "your eyes are bigger than your stomach," but have you ever thought that maybe it's really your bowl and plate that's bigger than your stomach? People unconsciously make a decision to eat more food from larger, lighter-colored dishes. However, you can slow your appetite down by going smaller and darker.

> **FACT:** Studies show that you will eat up to 50 to 70 percent less from smaller, darker blue- or gray-colored dishes.

The smaller sizes fool you into thinking you are eating a full-size meal, while the darker colors help suppress your appetite. Other than blueberries, there aren't too many appetizing foods that are dark blue or gray.

Choose to go on a fun shopping trip for new diet-friendly dishes! Make it an extra special trip by donating your current dishes to a family in need.

## MOM'S BRIGHT BITE

"I ate the whole thing!" is not something to celebrate. Successful dieting requires you to place *mind over platter*!

## 4. LET ME COACH YOU TO MAXIMIZE
## YOUR RESULTS USING MY
## ONLINE DIET MANAGEMENT PROGRAM.

Getting your waistline in-line is easier with my online weight loss management program at **www.RevivalDiet.com.**

I can help you achieve maximum diet and beauty results by encouraging you to be more persistent and consistent. I can be your virtual personal trainer and mom can be your personal cheerleader (pom-poms not included).

---

**FACT:** I'll still be tough on you and tell you
the truth, so don't expect a cake walk.

---

Revival's online program allows you to confidentially track your weight-loss progress online, plan and rotate your daily eating pattern, meet supportive friends, discuss hot topics on our message boards, receive encouraging e-mail reminders, keep a food diary, develop a walking/exercise plan, and more. You can also sign up for my free weight-loss newsletter and weight-loss blog for the latest diet with beauty and medical research breakthroughs.

Don't be like Jackie Gleason, who said, "The second day of a diet is always easier than the first. By the second day you're off it." Our online community helps you to keep your diet boots on and moving.

## 5. DON'T HIDE YOUR UNHEALTHY
## SNACK FOODS . . . THROW THEM AWAY!

You've probably been advised in the past to hide all food from your sight, particularly unhealthy snacks and junk food that puts the "junk in your trunk."

That's good advice based on good science—studies show that just *seeing* snack food results in huge binge eating. So hiding the bad food is a good idea, but throwing the bad food away is a great idea.

> **FACT:** Any food that is too unhealthy to
> keep on your countertop should be t
> hrown away, not hidden in your cabinets.

Let's be honest, putting the potato chips and cupcakes in the cabinet only makes you think about the potato chips and cupcakes still in those dark recesses. Ever taken a peek just to make sure they are in there by cracking open the cabinet door?

Just throw it all away—do it now while you are strong. Take a deep breath, put this book down right now, and just go do it. No crying or whining. It's time to exorcise the junk-food demons from your kitchen. Throw your family's snacks away, not your family!

As you are throwing the jelly doughnuts in the trashcan, I want you to think about how great you are going to look and feel soon. Pour out the sugary soft drinks that are making your *gluteus maximus* bigger than Rhode Island, while devastating your blood sugar health. Sugar drinks taste good to the last drop until they make your body drop to the ground.

For every item of junk food you throw away, reward yourself with something healthy in its place. So throw out the potato chips and replace them with crispy soy protein chips. Buy flavored no-calorie water or unsweetened teas in exchange for those super-sweet soft drinks. Choose foods you can be proud of, not foods you have to shamefully hide in the back corners of your pantry. Imagine mom and I visiting you to give your kitchen a medical checkup. What disease-causing foods would we find? Get rid of them to rescue yourself!

---

## MOM'S BRIGHT BITE

"How can I go on a diet? My cabinets are still full!"

Umm . . . no. There is no excuse for not taking action. If you can't stand the heat, run out of the kitchen.

---

## 6. POST UP YOUR "MOST-WANTED FOOD ENEMIES" LIST.

Take a sticky note (or sheet of paper) and write in big letters across the top: **Wanted for Attempted Murder of [Your Name]: Armed And Dangerous!**

Number and list the top three foods that are your worst enemies, then post it up on your mirror or refrigerator where you can clearly see it every morning and night.

In case you are curious, here's my list:

**Wanted for Attempted Murder of Aaron Tabor: Armed And Dangerous!**

1. Pizza
2. Sour candies
3. Chicken Alfredo

Since clearly listing these foods and posting them where I can see them, I've had amazing success at eating them in moderation.

---

**FACT:** Clearly naming your worst enemies—the ones that are making you ugly, fat, and killing you—forces you to make smarter "win" eating decisions.

---

Taste makes waist—choose to identify and see your food enemies clearly. Update your list from time to time as you become successful in beating certain enemy foods. Keep emergency food substitutes for your worst enemies handy to neutralize unexpected craving ambushes. Find lower fat, lower calorie versions of what you already love.

Many people are ambushed by between-meal and nighttime snacking attacks. Keeping Revival snacks onhand is the perfect countermeasure serving as your fat defense shield. *The Revival Slim & Beautiful Diet* gives you plenty of satisfying snack-substitution options. Other great snack examples include low-fat yogurt mixed with fruit and nuts, or low-fat, high-nutrition oatmeal.

---

### MOM'S BRIGHT BITE

Don't be like the dieter who said, "I gave up desserts! And, it was the worst twenty minutes of my life." Finding the right delicious snacks, like Revival's protein-packed snacks, makes your life tastier than ever—not tasteless torture.

---

## 7. WEIGH AND MEASURE ONCE WEEKLY.

As the tried-and-true business adage goes, "You can't manage what you can't measure." Measuring your weight-loss progress is critical because it will actually motivate you to succeed faster.

---

**FACT:** Monitoring your weight-loss productivity will increase your weight-loss productivity.

---

Each small step will make the next small step seem not only possible, but more probable. So, pick up a reliable scale and tape measure as soon as possible (more sweet shopping), and start using them. Keep a simple record of your weekly weight loss and decrease in waist circumference (as measured across your belly button). Track your results online as part of my web-based diet program, or write it down using this simple table.

DATE                    MY WEIGHT AND WAISTLINE

Starting Weight and Waistline: _____        _____

Week 1:                  _____        _____

Week 2:                  _____        _____

Week 3:                  _____        _____

Week 4:                  _____        _____

Week 5:                  _____        _____

Week 6:                  _____        _____

Week 7:                  _____        _____

Week 8:                  _____        _____

Week 9:                  _____        _____

Week 10:                 _____        _____

Week 11:                 _____        _____

Week 12:                 _____        _____

Week 13:                 _____        _____

Week 14:                 _____        _____

Week 15:                 _____        _____

Week 16:                 _____        _____

I *do not* recommend weighing or measuring every day, because day-to-day water weight and circumference fluctuations can incorrectly discourage you. Your weekly downward trends are the only important measurements. I weigh and measure on Sunday nights because it motivates me to not blow my diet on Friday and Saturday, when everyone wants to eat huge amounts of food.

Choose to motivate yourself by regularly measuring your progress.

P.S. Remember to share your weekly weight loss success with your Diet Buddy "competitor." Make it your goal to lose more weekly than your Diet Buddy!

---

## MOM'S BRIGHT BITE

### How to Use a Weight Scale Properly
Follow these hilarious rules for your best weight-loss results:

1. Before weighing yourself, calibrate your scale properly by turning the little round knob so that the scale's needle is as far to the left of zero pounds as possible. Note: avoid digital scales because they can't be calibrated properly.
2. Remove all clothing, jewelry, and false teeth (or any other removable parts), use the bathroom, and dry your hair thoroughly (preferably, cut your hair first).
3. Hold tightly onto the sink and towel bar (both if possible) and gradually release the weight of your body onto the scale with caution.
4. Place only one foot on the scale and hang a couple of toes over the side against the floor for better stabilization.
5. Immediately stop lowering yourself if you experience emotional discomfort, or if the needle rapidly approaches 130 pounds.
6. Do not weigh yourself more than once yearly because each use of the scale damages the little springs inside, thus making you appear to weigh more each time.

7. Buy a scale from a store with a 100 percent money back guarantee. Return scale for repair if you notice any weight gain over time.

And to settle the issue once and for all, the scales in your doctor's office are always wrong!

## 8. PERFECT AND PROTECT YOUR DIET RESULTS AND BEAUTY WITH THE RIGHT VITAMINS, MINERALS, ANTIOXIDANTS, AND BEAUTY SUPPLEMENTS.

Choosing to take the proper dietary supplements gives your body the extra beauty perfection and protection it deserves. It's your daily decision. Mom and I believe our health and beauty are worth it.

The right dietary supplement can protect your body from nutritional deficiencies during weight loss. Antioxidants help neutralize unhealthy free radicals. Bone-healthy calcium may help you keep your weight under control. Recent studies suggest that calcium and dairy foods may lessen hunger.

**FACT:** In addition to the soy protein and soy antioxidants documented by my team, other scientists have discovered new beauty ingredients—including marine *glycosaminoglycans*, peptides, amino acids, and seed extracts—that produce dramatic positive effects on the appearance of skin, hair, and nails.

You choose to perfect-and-protect the appearance of your skin, hair, and nails with the right dietary ingredients. New beauty research breakthroughs on "beauty from within" dietary supplement ingredients are remarkable. With the new ingredients being discovered, you can actually perfect your beauty, instead of just protecting it.

Of course, using the proper ingredients is necessary for good health. Because this is such an important part of your total-body beauty and diet results, I've formulated a comprehensive "Gorgeous Roses" dietary supplement to eliminate the guesswork and confusion while maximizing beauty results for your "rose petals and stems." Making sure the latest ingredients and research technology are incorporated into the formula is a priority.

My expert nutrition staff can help you select the perfect beauty and diet nutritional makeover supplement by calling **1-800-REVIVAL** (1-800-738-4825), visiting **www.RevivalDiet.com** or e-mailing **Nutrition@RevivalDiet.com**.

Choose to perfect your beauty diet results with the right beauty dietary supplements.

## 9. YOUR MOM WAS RIGHT: NEVER, EVER SKIP BREAKFAST!

It's 8:00 p.m. The kids are in bed. You're eating a bowl of ice cream and surfing the Internet. It's 11:00 p.m. You fall asleep. At 7:00 a.m. the alarm rings. You get up, shower, dress, wake the kids, dress them, feed them and by 8:30, you're out the door. You were so busy taking care of your family that you didn't have time to eat for yourself. By 9:00 a.m. you are at the office and getting prepared for your weekly staff meeting.

What's wrong with this scenario? For thirteen hours, your body has been fasting. How can you expect to run efficiently throughout the day if you haven't fueled up? You wouldn't expect to take a road trip with your car running on empty.

When you go without eating for an extended period of time, your brain reacts by sending signals to the body that you are starving, and your metabolism slows to conserve energy. Then when you finally eat again, the body thinks it needs to reserve energy in preparation for more food deprivation.

Therefore it stores calories in the form of fat. So, *not* eating can actually lead to weight gain.

---

**FACT:** Some people think that they actually eat more on the days they consume a morning meal than on days that they don't eat. However, a recent research study debunks this belief. Skipping breakfast causes you to eat more calories.

---

Studies have also shown that people who eat breakfast eat more nutrients and less fat and cholesterol, are less likely to be overweight, have more energy and better concentration throughout the day, and have healthier cholesterol levels.

Eating breakfast every day places you on the downward weight-loss path. On the *Revival Slim and Beautiful Diet* plan you can start your day with protein-packed Revival bars and shakes. Add fruit for the extra energy and antioxidants.

Choose to feel fuller longer by eating breakfast regularly. Dodge the doughnuts, croissants, and high-sugar cereals: A moment on the lips, a lifetime on the hips!

---

## MOM'S BRIGHT BITE

Do you know the two things you should never eat before breakfast? Lunch and dinner! Breakfast is just that . . . breaking a fast. Those great pastries and goodies at work or church are not the best way to get your blood sugar levels back! Try low-glycemic options to prevent the spike-crash-burn events.

---

## 10. COLD WATER = COOL WAIST AND BRIGHT FACE.

Drinking ice-cold, calorie-free water is a great way to help warm up your weight loss results. Why? Your body has to burn calories to warm up the cold water to your core body temperature (98.6 degrees).

---

**FACT:** You burn approximately 7 calories per cup of ice-cold fluid. If that doesn't sound like much, multiply that times 8 to 12 glasses per day, then times 30 days per month, and then times 12 months to burn 6 to 9 pounds worth of calories per year.

---

Drinking lots of water not only reduces your appetite by simply filling you up, but it is also very important for keeping your skin hydrated (just think about dehydrated lettuce to visualize the importance of water to your skin) and your body energized.

---

### MOM'S BRIGHT BITE

Finally, some "just desserts" for the unscrupulous men out there!

Two blond men decided to split a can of diet soda. One blond opened the can, and poured half the contents into his own glass and half into his friend's glass. Before tossing the can, he stopped to read the nutritional information on the side.

"Only one calorie per can," he read aloud.

"Hmm," murmured the other blond. "I wonder which glass has the calorie?"

---

Reach for ultra-pure bottled water instead of spring water, because it is cleaner and healthier without toxins or inorganic matter. Drink unsweetened tea (green or black) or liposomal powered beauty water for extra antioxidant benefits.

Choose to give fat the cold shoulder by drinking ice-cold water (or other calorie-free fluids like flavored water).

P.S. Have some fun by asking your waiter for "ice-cold diet water"—you will be amused by the puzzled looks you will receive.

## 11. HUNGRY FOR SOME SLEEP?
## GET YOUR SLEEP TO STAY SKINNY.

Sleep puts the beauty in Sleeping Beauty.

Feeling (and looking) overworked, overscheduled, and overweight? Most of us can raise our hand high to this question. Sleep deprivation harms your weight, energy level, and skin, hair, and nail appearance.

> **FACT:** Lack of sleep makes you moody, depressed, and anxious, which can lead to overeating. Also, our skin, hair, and nails repair best during the night, so lack of sleep diminishes your beauty's natural regeneration ability.

Why does lack of sleep cause weight gain? We have some clues.

Shortage of sleep lowers levels of a hormone that suppresses the appetite—for the intellectually curious, the hormone is called *leptin*—making you feel hungry. Shortage of sleep also raises levels of another hormone—*ghrelin*—that causes you to feel hungry. It's a lose-lose eating situation.

So, here are some practical suggestions for getting a good night's sleep. Try to relax before going to bed—a hot bath surrounded by lit soy candles (which burn without forming carcinogens!) followed by stretching is the perfect "bedtime story."

Avoid spicy foods and late meals. Avoid caffeine especially later in the day (no caffeine after 4:00 p.m.). Try Revival's caffeine-free roasted soybean "coffee" alone or blended with real coffee for caffeine-free or reduced caffeine options.

Check drugs and supplements for their suggested intake times. Some herbs and medications, such as decongestants, can increase the heart rate or activate brain activity, making it difficult to sleep.

Choose to reduce your hunger by getting seven to nine hours of sleep per night. Don't just dream about a full night's sleep—make it happen! You may need to rearrange your life to be on a more consistent sleep schedule. Your health is well worth the effort it takes.

## 12. WALK THIS WAY FOR A SKINNY BODY, SUPER ENERGY, AND SUNNY MOOD.

Winning the "Employee of the Month" parking spot is not a reward for your waistline. I know you are thinking, "Oh great, another exercise speech" after I've already covered the importance of walking as part of the diet and physical activity plan. I've chosen to retouch on it here to emphasize its importance to your overall health. It is going to make you feel good.

> **FACT:** Regular exercise is just as powerful as common anti-depressant medications in boosting your mood. This creates a positive feedback loop—the more you exercise, the better you feel, so the less you eat.

Ever noticed the warning labels on stationary exercise bikes? *Discontinue use if you feel shortness of breath or experience discomfort when using this equipment.*

Many of us have taken it literally by simply never exercising again because we felt discomfort the last time we attempted to start an exercise program—so we simply became couch potatoes!

Was "No pain, No gain" running through your mind for a brief five seconds before you "discontinued use" of your body and dreams for life? Well, try this health headline on for size: "Good News: No Hurt Required to Lose!"

Walking is the perfect low-impact, enjoyable solution. Don't show ingratitude for your ability to walk by making excuses. It's easy to start a walking program and it doesn't hurt! A brisk walk during lunch is a great way to boost your metabolism and mood. Make it brisk, baby!

For maximum diet and beauty results choose to walk at least six days a week for at least thirty to forty-five minutes. Too busy for a full thirty-to-forty-five minute walk all at once? Try several ten-minute power walks, spaced throughout your day, to keep your energy up and to lower your blood pressure.

## MOM'S BRIGHT BITE

You know it is time to start a regular walking program if you find certain body parts refusing to leave the floor when you try to do a few push ups, even when you are on your knees leaning forward!

Take your walking from great to best by asking your Diet Buddy and/or family to walk with you for some great talk time. Kids and grandkids will also love the adventure, and they will likely keep you moving at a faster pace to burn more calories.

Be young and cool—buy an iPod to listen to your favorite "make me fit" music while you walk (make sure you download "Rescue Me" by Fontella Bass). Listening to music from your earlier years will energize your walk! *Feel eighteen again.*

**FACT:** Walking is the easiest way to start something good, but it's just the beginning of your path. Before long, you will find yourself with an urge to pick up your pace—and maybe even start running or lifting weights. You may even get around to taking those dance lessons with your spouse that you never started!

Good walking or running shoes with a great arch support are a must—so grab some new shoes if yours don't have firm arch support. Make it a healthier shopping trip by walking briskly and taking the stairs. Light stretching before and after you walk will make your muscles feel great and put a smile on your face. Too rainy or too cold? Head to your local mall or walk in place at home with the tunes blasting.

If you find yourself too undisciplined to exercise, at least be smart enough to do something about it! Join my online diet management program at **www.RevivalDiet.com** or hire a personal trainer if you can afford one. A step counter (also called a pedometer) is an electronic device clipped to your belt that automatically measures your steps (can be purchased online or at any fitness store). Start a daily total steps competition with your Diet Buddy.

You will also find the single most effective exercise for toning your sagging *gluteus maximus* (and other troublesome spots) at the Revival Web site!

## MOM'S BRIGHT BITE

Two things are certain in this life . . . death and taxes. Don't tax your health to death with a poor diet and lack of exercise.

## 13. DE-STRESS FOR LESS . . . LESS POUNDS.

Stress helps makes you fat and unhealthy. Period. Some scientists estimate that 75 to 90 percent of all doctor visits are related to stress.

---

**FACT:** Stress causes you to store more food as ugly belly fat.

---

How? Unchecked stress levels increase stress hormone levels (like cortisol). Long-term consequences of uncontrolled stress include a very dirty laundry list:

- Overeating, leading to excessive fat
- Poor skin
- Headaches
- Poor memory
- Hypothyroidism
- Ulcers and other digestive problems
- High blood pressure
- Chest pains
- Fatigue
- Depression
- Diabetes
- Decreased muscle tissue
- Bone loss
- Poor immune function
- Anxiety
- Sleep disorders

Wow! I don't know about you, but it stressed me out just reading the list. Choose to stress less by identifying the cause(s) of your stress and then taking immediate action to re-shape your life.

Your health is too important to succumb to stress. Life is short enough already.

Here are some easy stress-reducing strategies:

- Strategize rather than stew about what's causing your stress. Instead of letting stress kidnap your emotions, take control by making a "Most Wanted Stress Enemies" list. Carefully consider what you can do to either a) change circumstances that would relieve your stress, or b) adjust your attitude so it won't sabotage your thoughts. Curing the stress-causing problems is better than applying a bandage, so make an intense effort to fix them and forget them.
- Play your favorite music every day to soothe your soul.
- Get plenty of sleep—a tired mind is a troubled mind.
- Find a trusted friend to share your thoughts and emotions.
- Seek professional and spiritual help if your stress is severe.

---

### MOM'S BRIGHT BITE

Beware: "stressed" is "desserts" spelled backward!

---

## 14. CHECKUP INSTEAD OF CHECKING OUT!

I recommend a complete physical exam every year for everyone of all ages, and particularly before starting a weight-loss program.

A good physical exam at least once every twelve months can save your life, through early detection of deadly diseases like cancer or heart disease. It can also detect medical conditions that could be packing pounds on your body.

**FACT:** Rapid weight gain, or difficulty in losing weight,
could both be due to low thyroid hormone levels
(a condition called *hypothyroidism*) or other
medical disorders. Nearly 10 percent of people
suffer from hypothyroidism, so make sure your doctor
checks for it, along with testing your cholesterol levels.

Hypothyroidism is an under-active thyroid, meaning that not enough of the thyroid hormone is being produced by your thyroid gland (located near the front of your neck). This imbalance has a direct effect on the rate your body burns calories, and your heart rate and body temperature.

Weight gain, fatigue, muscle weakness or pain, increased blood cholesterol, dry, pale, or puffy skin, depression, constipation, and/or heavier menstrual periods could all be symptoms of hypothyroidism.

Choose a check-up to help you check-out the extra pounds safely and effectively. Ask your doctor to check for hypothyroidism and other medical conditions that could be causing persistent weight gain.

## 15. THE CULINARY KITCHEN SINK: EVERY COMMON-SENSE PIECE OF EATING ADVICE YOUR MOM TOLD YOU . . . AND MORE.

Hey, it never hurts to review—even if we have already heard these at least a hundred times. It only hurts if we don't follow this advice.

- *Eat smaller portions.* Eat smaller to be smaller. The key to enjoying smaller portion sizes is learning to savor each bite (you are an adult now, you know, and you can control your swallowing reflex). Practice deriving as much pleasure as possible from each bite of a smaller portion size. Apply the same to snacks and desserts: indulge in a smaller piece of chocolate by letting it slowly melt in your mouth to tease your taste buds. Get the picture? Good things do come in smaller packages!

---

### MOM'S BRIGHT BITE

Many people blow up their waistline by having romantic dinners for two . . . *alone!* Stuffing too much food into our tummies will quickly make our rear ends look like five pounds of sausage stuffed into a two-pound sack! I knew it was time to take action when it felt like my long-line waist-cincher was cracking my ribs during a deep breath.

---

- *Never skip meals* because your body will think it's starving. It kicks into survival mode. Your metabolism slows to conserve energy. Then when you eat again, the body stores calories as fat in preparation of future food deprivation.

---

### MOM'S BRIGHT BITE

Lose weight by skipping . . . junk food, unhealthy snacks, and dessert.

---

- *"Don't eat your food so fast!"* We've all heard mom yell these words across the table. You will be pleasantly surprised at how quickly you feel full when you eat slowly. Doing so allows your mind to catch up with your stomach to prevent excessive calorie consumption. We've all stuffed down too much sweet or fatty food too fast, only to suffer the consequences later. Wait for the pleasure to hit you from the first three bites of a sweet food instead of eating all six donuts at once. Eat slowly, eat guilt-free, and savor each bite to win the fat fight.

## MOM'S BRIGHT BITE

Doctors say that if you eat slowly, you will eat less . . . particularly if you are a member of a large family.

- *Pack in the protein* to reduce hunger. Protein sends "I'm full!" messages from your stomach to your brain to keep you satisfied longer.
- *Eat antioxidant rich fruits and vegetables* for healthier skin and tissues. The easy-to-remember rule: enjoy five or more servings of three different colors daily. Don't overload vegetables with butter and salt—in moderation there is minimization of your waistline.
- *Reduce refined, simple carbs* like sweets, soda pop, white bread, and alcohol. Simple carbs cause high blood-sugar levels. Consequently, insulin is over-secreted by your body, causing some excess blood sugar to be stored as fat.

## MOM'S BRIGHT BITE

The most fattening thing you can put in an ice-cream sundae is a spoon! Have you bought your smaller bowls and plates yet?

- *Increase complex carbs* (i.e., smart-carbs or foods with a low-glycemic index) because they don't cause rapid increases in blood-sugar levels. Protein-packed foods, reduced-fat dairy products, beans, rice, pasta, whole-grain bread, potatoes, and corn contain complex carbohydrates. Most Revival products have a clinically proven low-glycemic index.
- *Be "smart" by enjoying Revival protein-packed soy pasta!* A recent clinical trial documented that Revival protein-packed soy pasta is a smart-carb,

meaning it won't cause a rapid rise in blood-sugar levels like simple carbs do. And, with eight grams of heart-healthy, energizing soy protein (14 grams total protein), dieters have a big reason to smile.

- *Reduce your overall fat intake* by reading labels. Moderate fat intake is not bad—it keeps your skin and nerve cell membranes healthy. Reach for olive oil for additional beauty and health benefits. Avoid killer "*trans* fats" completely because even small amounts can kill you. (*Trans* fats are now clearly labeled in the nutrition facts, so just look on the food label!)

---

## MOM'S BRIGHT BITE

"I only overeat chocolate for you, so there will be more of me to love" is not an acceptable excuse!

---

- *Get your fiber* with at least 25 to 30 grams of soluble fiber a day. Foods high in soluble fiber include oatmeal, beans, peas, rice, bran, barley, citrus fruits, strawberries, and apples. Fiber helps you feel fuller longer and supports better digestive-tract function.
- *Coffee and caffeine* are fine to enjoy unless you experience negative side effects, including nervousness or irritability, trouble in sleeping, dizziness, or a fast or pounding heartbeat. Avoid high-calorie coffee loaded with fattening cream; instead, try iced coffee with skim milk or nonfat cream instead.

---

**FACT:** Putting the *Fifteen Physical Laws of Accelerated Weight Loss* into practice will help you "arrest and prosecute" felonious fat in its tracks.

---

Choose to accelerate and maximize your weight-loss results.

---

## MOM'S BRIGHT BITE

### Seven Diet Laws NOT to Live By

1. Candy has zero calories if you don't tell your Diet Buddy about it.
2. Drink a diet soda while eating a candy bar, so the calories in the candy bar are canceled out by the lack of calories in the diet soda.
3. Look thinner by fattening up all of your family, friends, and co-workers!
4. Drink a milkshake before each meal to take the edge off your appetite so you will eat less.
5. Eat food with as many preservatives as possible to preserve your age and looks.
6. Instead of acknowledging you are fat and doing something about it, just keep on believing you are just short for your weight.
7. Food that doesn't taste great has zero calories, so just go ahead and finish devouring that mediocre pastry at your office breakfast.

---

## CHAPTER 6

# Put A Tiger In Your Tank . . . Energize Me!

*Energy and persistence alter all things.*
—Benjamin Franklin

*During the first week of using Revival, I noticed my energy level soaring especially in the afternoons.*

—M. Schroeder, Results not typical.[†]

*My energy has more than doubled with Revival.*

—B. Baumer, Results not typical.[†]

*I no longer experience the 'mid-morning slump' . . .*

—M. R. Carlisle, Results not typical.[†]

*The most noticeable benefit was my increase in energy level and my weight loss. Many people notice my energy level and they want to know, "What are you on?" I'm constantly telling people about Revival because the products taste great and they make me feel great too.*

—Y. Castillo, Results not typical.[†]

---

[†]Results not typical, but included to motivate you. Individual results vary. You must follow the calorie-restricted diet plan, physical activity plan, and dietary supplement regimens presented in this book if you hope to achieve great weight loss, beauty, and health results. see *Introduction* and specific studies presented in this book for typical results. These statements have not been evaluated by the Food and Drug Administration. Revival is not intended to diagnose, treat, cure, or prevent any disease.

## DO YOUR ENERGY LEVELS MAKE OTHERS
## ASK YOU, "WHAT ARE YOU ON?"

Well, they will. Wake up and get ready to roll because this chapter is a ten-minute, short, sweet, and intense boot camp on increasing your energy.

So polish up those diet boots—double-speed—and stay close behind me. I'm going to share with you "The Four Gospels of Gorgeous Energy!" Mom and I have found four simple, doable truths to turn the timid kitty in your tank into a tenacious tiger.

---

**FACT**: High energy will empower you
to win your nutritional war.

---

Are you following me? Soaring physical energy not only feels great, but it also energizes your spirit and willpower to take the persistent steps needed for altering your looks and your life. In other words, great energy will help make you gorgeous.

Let's see how energizing the truth can be!

---

### MOM'S BRIGHT BITE

Most of us relate to Winnie the Pooh, forever in search of a little "smackerel" to eat—something energizing from Rabbit's "hunny" pot. Or maybe you relate to the droopy-eared Eeyore who appears to have woken up only to daydream of going to sleep again. But do you wonder what it would be like to be one of *those* people, the Tiggers of this world, who bounce out of bed eager to walk, run, work, play, and joyfully pester other people to do the same?

---

Well, take heart. There is a Tigger in your tank just waiting to bounce and bounce and bounce—all you need are the right treats to lure him out!

## THE FOUR GOSPELS OF GORGEOUS ENERGY

*Eat, Drink, Sleep, and Be Merry for today our energy will rise!*
—Doc and Mom

### Gospel #1: Eat to Beat an Energy Defeat!

Bored out of your mind with monotonous energy levels? I know—it's time for a change.

You can bite your way into eternal energy bliss with low-glycemic choices instead of tormenting your body (and looks) on a sickening high-glycemic roller-coaster ride. High-glycemic foods quickly push sugar into your bloodstream, causing a sugar spike followed by a screaming race downward. It isn't a sweet feeling!

Eating high-glycemic foods is like riding a dietary rollercoaster to the tallest peak, sailing over the tip in near weightlessness, and then plunging downward, forced into your seat at a stomach-sickening pace. Imagine doing that over and over—for hours, days, weeks, months, and years. It takes a huge toll on your health and can change your once adorable pancreas into an ugly duckling that will never grow up.

The race down makes you crave more food and traps you in a vicious cycle (We've all filled our shopping carts up with junk by making the mistake of shopping for groceries while hungry—dumb idea). By the time you make it to the end of the ride, you are exhausted from all of the sugary excitement you can stand. We've all seen kids gorge themselves with candy, go absolutely berserk for an hour, and then crash like baby bears hibernating for the winter. As adults, we just push ahead more tired than ever without the kindergarten luxury of 1:00 p.m. naptime.

---

**FACT:** Dietary amusement park rides
that drain your energy aren't any fun.

---

The worst high-glycemic foods you can ride include sweets, soda pops, white bread, and alcohol.

On the other hand (or I should say, "in the other hand"), low-glycemic choices, also called smart-carbs, slowly release energy to your body. It feels like an eternal energy supply compared to the fleeting thrill of high-glycemic foods. Your sugar levels rise up slow and low with a gentle ride back down. It's a walk in the park for your body and blood sugar, instead of a scream-filled roller-coaster race.

The best low-glycemic food rides not to miss include protein, reduced-fat dairy products, beans, rice, pasta, whole grain bread, potatoes, and corn. The best way to easily benefit from low-glycemic energy is to reach for protein-packed Revival bars, shakes, pasta, and other products.

A recent Revival human clinical trial, with the glycemic index experts down under at the University of Sydney in Australia, found that Revival soy protein bars, shakes, pasta, protein chips, and soy nuts do not cause a rapid rise in blood sugar like regular "dumb" sugars do. Your pancreas has an adorable smile just from looking at this graph!

So now I understand why mom has the energy of a lab rat on caffeine when she eats Revival. She says it is good to have bundles of energy when she has to help manage a busy company *and* comb as much hair as she has now.

The benefits of protein-packed foods don't just end with a low-glycemic index. Protein is a great source of energy itself. Revival milk-protein-based products and soy-protein-based products also supply branched-chain

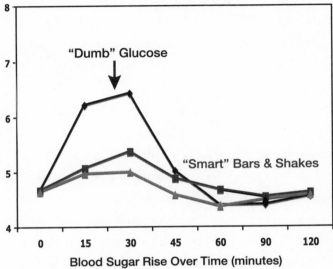

Clinically Proven Low-Glycemic Index for Revival Soy

amino acids that can be burned by your body to produce energy and to help build lean muscle mass.

A multivitamin rich in the B-complex vitamins and Coenzyme Q10 (which nourishes your "energy factories" in every cell) is the perfect sidekick for additional energy support. You can stay up-to-date on the latest energy dietary supplements by contacting my friendly nutrition staff for expert advice at **1-800-REVIVAL** (1-800-738-4825), **www.RevivalDiet.com**, or **Nutrition@RevivalDiet.com**.

Listen to a few more Revival-LITES talk about the joy of low-glycemic, energizing dietary choices:

*My chiropractor recommended Revival. The main benefit is the leanness of my body. I lift weights, run, and do power yoga, and I can really notice the change in my body shape and muscular development. I am pleased with the results. I have noticed a difference in my skin—it looks and feels healthier, and people comment on it. I modified my diet to eliminate high-glycemic foods. Now I have more energy and stamina. I have a general sense of well-being. I am positive Revival benefits me tremendously as part of my whole regimen. I continue to take Revival and will plan to do so for the rest of my life. I believe in your product and am so grateful for it. I have compared the ingredients of Revival with competitors and you always come out on top!*

—L. Phillips, Results not typical.[†]

*Aloha! I am enjoying Revival. During the past three to four weeks, I have noticed a dramatic increase in energy and vitality whenever I have Revival. By using Revival and my current fitness program, I can surely say that I am on my way to a leaner and much more fit body than I could have ever expected. Thank you Revival Family for the products and information that are so vital in helping me to finally have the body that I have always dreamed of having!"*

—B. Dahlig, Results not typical.[†]

Choose to be smart, and don't drive a spike in the heart of your energy levels by splurging on dumb sugar foods. You can choose to soar with protein-packed, low-glycemic soy protein products instead. When you eat right, you will defeat wrong.

Recognize when your energy is falling (typically mid-morning and mid-afternoon) and reach for another protein-packed treat to keep feeding your energy. Your tenacious tiger will jump through hoops for protein-packed, low-glycemic treats.

Did you think you were really going to escape this chapter without me telling you that breakfast is *critical* for getting all-day energy levels off to the right start? Consider this your warning ticket, served with a protein-packed court date within thirty minutes of waking—don't wait two hours to eat!

For more details on specific low-glycemic and high-glycemic foods, slow down and stop by for a visit at **www.RevivalDiet.com**.

## MOM'S BRIGHT BITE

One of my friends told me she couldn't afford to work out any more because her health club charged $60 per workout session. Startled, I asked if that included a free massage, too!

"No," she said, "I paid $60 for a two-month membership, but only went once!"

Well, mystery solved. Eating protein-packed, low-glycemic foods can help you have enough energy to work out in the first place. Working out will then create more energy. Energy is truly the gift that keeps on giving.

A daily walking program and lifting some small weights at home is free and fun. When I walk, I love the extra time to think about my day, say a prayer, and plan for the future. I'll save my $60 for a new, smaller dress.

### Gospel #2: Drink Up to Turn Water Into Your Energy Miracle!

Drink, drink, and drink when you are feeling tired. Filling up on fluids will make you more alert and puts energy in your tank. Let me show you why.

**FACT:** You can pump up your energy levels by filling up with lots of fluids. You will find it impossible to sit still when you're drinking enough ice-cold fluids daily.

You know how it feels to be mildly dehydrated after a hot day in the sun, a hard day shopping, or an illness—it feels awful to be de-energized. Mild dehydration can produce headaches, muscle aches, back pain, and a lack of energy. As you get older, you start losing your thirst sensitivity fine-tuning, so you can become mildly dehydrated without even realizing it! While you can't actually turn calorie-free fluids like water into energy (that *would* be a miracle), drinking eight to twelve ice-cold glasses a day can help you burn calories, hydrate your skin, muscles, and achy joints, and make you feel fully ready to take on today's challenges.

So don't sit around being a deadhead, just drink and drink and drink. If you were a plant, I would water you myself. But fortunately, you can use your own brain to think and drink.

If you don't have regular access to ice-cold water or other fluids, carry a little bottle in your purse or briefcase. There's no excuse to not drink enough daily. Drink ultra-purified water, if possible, to avoid toxins and high levels of inorganic matter found in typical spring and tap waters. Sip antioxidant-rich tea (green or black) for extra skin and health benefits. I'm currently developing a new beauty water with liposomes containing skin- and body-energizing vitamins, minerals, and antioxidants.

Caffeine can be a powerful ally if walked on a short leash. Teas will give you some caffeine, but lap up more concentrated caffeinated fluids for an uplifting energy burst. Try iced-coffee with skim milk for low calories and some extra calcium. Consume caffeine in moderation—if Starbucks contacts you about being their official mascot, or if you can't remember the last time you blinked, you've had way too much caffeine. If you use exclamation points almost every sentence, you've had way too much caffeine! And no, coffee beans are not vegetables either!

Choose to put a hydrated spring in your step. In fact, why don't you stop for a water break right now? Your tenacious tiger will swim laps around tired teenagers when watered generously.

## Gospel #3: Sleep Deep to Make Sweet Energy Dreams Your Reality.

You energy's worst enemy is sleep deprivation. So, hit the hay. Grab some shut-eye. Rack up. Crawl in. Kip down. Sack out. Turn in. Retire. It doesn't matter how you say it—just get more of it! Snuggle up with seven to nine hours of the good stuff nightly, or you will wake up one day to find your beauty and health gone. Just take a look at your eyes after one bad night's rest and imagine what is also happening inside your body, too.

---

**FACT:** Even if you think you are getting enough sleep, you are probably not getting enough high-quality sleep during the right time frame.

---

As my granddad used to tell me, "An hour's sleep before midnight is worth two after midnight." Getting eight hours of sleep from 2:00 a.m. to 10:00 a.m. is not the same quality as getting eight hours of sleep from 10:00 p.m. to 6:00 a.m. We all know exactly how poor a poor night's rest makes us look and feel.

Did you know that some studies even suggest working a night shift job increases cancer risk? Our bodies were designed to sleep when it is dark and work when it is light. Altering a built-in biological fact isn't healthy. Don't sleep walk through life. Make drastic changes to your lifestyle—just fix it now!

There are bonus rewards for the well rested: a good night's sleep is the cheapest makeover you can get and an inexpensive alternative to plastic surgery for puffy, dark circles under your eyes. Your skin cells divide and reproduce the fastest around 11:00 p.m. every night, so being in bed *asleep* by then, not watching a home shopping channel or reading a diet book, helps nurture your natural beauty renewal process.

Since counting sheep isn't proven to help you overcome difficulty falling asleep, try relaxing with a hot bath and carcinogen-free soy candles. Trade relaxing face and neck massages with your spouse. If night sweats from menopause are keeping you up, eat a Revival soy bar or shake. Of course, avoid the late-night caffeine, spicy foods, meals, or herbs and drugs that may keep you awake. Completely darkening your bedroom at night may work wonders—it certainly does for me. If all else fails, try a dietary-supplement sleep aid, like melatonin or valerian root, to help regulate your body clock. If you do finally run out of sheep to count, try a small dose of non-addictive prescription sleep medicine from your doctor as a last resort.

Choose to awaken to a world of wonders with extra energy. As mom says, "A good night's rest will make everything better in the morning." Your tenacious tiger will be frisky with fortitude when you get enough sleep.

### Gospel #4: Be Merry: Purposefully Create a Merry Spirit.

A merry mind doeth good, like a medicine for your energy.

Making a choice on a daily basis to *create* an energetic spirit is your most potent weapon to rule over your meek and weak old nature. Purposefully creating a merrier mind will lead the rest of your body into energy euphoria.

Give your tenacious tiger these seven energy-boosting treats to chew on every day:

1. *Let there be light!* As soon as possible after waking up, take in several big eyefuls of sunshine. It's a great time to pause and say thanks for another day. If it's dark or cloudy, turn on all of the lights in the room you are in, including all of the lights in your bathroom when you are getting ready in the morning. Buy extra lights, but don't forget to turn them off when you leave! Light is a powerful, positive drug to warm up your mind and energy. Don't underestimate its "triple-strength" effectiveness. Recharge with solar-power. Just remember: Light—it's what's for breakfast . . . and your mid-afternoon pick-me-up, too.

2. *Let there be music!* Even though music can tame the wild beast, the right music can put major tempo into your tenacious tiger. Use your favorite high-energy tunes to turn up your personal energy volume. Some rhythm makes every shower or bath better. (More

shopping is in order, this time for a small bathroom stereo system!) Earphones at work for your iPod or computer can whip up some wonders to beat those mid-afternoon valleys.

3. *Let there be stretching!* Even puppies and kittens know that a good stretch is the best way to start the morning. So shake the nighttime rust out of your joints, muscles, and mind to stretch your energy beyond its current limits. Applying a full-body moisturizer after a shower is the perfect way to stretch while saving your skin.

---

### MOM'S BRIGHT BITE

*You know you are getting old when the candles cost more than the cake.*
—BOB HOPE

"Old" is such a harsh word . . . I prefer to say "vintage"!

Let me tell you about my new best friend. Enjoying soy candles while soaking in the tub (usually at the end of a strenuous day) has quickly become one of my most anticipated simple pleasures. It's my time.

Lavender, mint, vanilla, and green gardenia are some of my favorite scents that I've formulated into long-burning soy candles, free of smoke or carcinogens.

---

4. *Let there be scents!* Ever wonder why most cleansers come in a lemon scent? Lemon makes you feel like working and cleaning. It was recognized decades ago that lemon increases productivity. Scents can help "stinking" energy levels smell more fragrant almost immediately. Burning the right aromatherapy candles (find a scent that works for you) or enjoying the right aromatherapy oils can create burning

energy inside of you. My on-call energy secret during medical school was lemon or peppermint tea bags that I kept in my scrubs' pocket for a quick sniff of sunshine.

5. *Let there be motion!* Physical motion puts your energy production in motion. So put your foot down and start walking to shout "no!" at low energy levels. Exercise is proven to boost your mood and metabolism (and burn calories), but you already knew that didn't you?

Jump up and down. Move your legs under your desk. Take the stairs. Park as far away as possible (without making yourself late). Walk!

Let your walking lead to brisk walking. Let your brisk walking lead to jogging or other low-impact aerobic exercise (like swimming). Let your aerobic exercise lead to lifting small weights (try two-pound dumbbells beside your weight scale). Let your small lifting lead to weight training. You may be laughing right now thinking of yourself lifting weights, but you never know how far your road will take you when you choose to use small steps to consistently win small battles time after time.

6. *Let there be laughter and smiles!* Laughter is not only great medicine, but it's also great tiger food. Need laughs? Sign up for a daily clean joke to be e-mailed to you from an online joke site. Search for "daily clean jokes" in your Internet search engine—try "vegetable jokes" if you are addicted to them after this book. Share the mirth with your Diet Buddy, Revival Diet Small Group, co-workers, friends, and family. Before long they will be tickling you back with jokes.

Smile. A lot. It sends a cue to your brain that something good is going on and perks up accordingly. Don't believe me? Try smiling while thinking of something sad, and then try frowning while thinking of something happy. Weird! Your brain is already trained to associate positive face *positions* with positive *emotions*. Smiling puts everyone around you in a better, more energetic mood. Create your positive environment with your words and facial posture. You are in control.

---

## MOM'S BRIGHT BITE

*Always laugh when you can. It is cheap medicine.*
—LORD BYRON

I was thrilled to read that laughter is so good for us that doctors sometimes call it *internal jogging*. If that is the case, my insides should be in wonderful condition!

One of my favorite humorists of all time is Erma Bombeck. Here's one of my favorite quotes from her that never fails to make me laugh out loud: "Seize the moment. Remember all those women on the Titanic who waved off the dessert cart."

It was also Erma who profoundly said: "If you can laugh at it, you can live with it."

I've learned over the years that laughter is one of God's most precious survival tools gifted to us. By choosing to see an aggravating or embarrassing situation through "Erma's eyes," I can quickly turn my lemons into laughter.

Don't forget to do some internal jogging today by choosing to run on the funny side of life's often-hilarious street. You can find fun in everyday challenges if you are looking. And above all else, enjoy a good hard laugh at yourself as often as possible.

---

7. *Let there be less stress!* Stress gobbles up your happy chemicals just like an elephant dispatches peanuts. An unhappy mind doesn't translate into an energetic body, so put a stop to it. Identify and

eliminate the cause of the stress instead of just putting a bandage over the symptoms.

Close your eyes and take a deep breath once in awhile. My grandmother says, "Just let all your worries rinse off your body and down the shower drain every day." She's eighty-five and still working because she likes it. She gets a massage every week. She told me to tell you that she highly recommends it because it relaxes her mind and energizes her spirit. My other grandmother is ninety and walks every day.

Refuse to ever stop.

Perfecting your energy utopia is so important that you should seek professional or spiritual help if needed, particularly if medical depression is causing your lack of energy.

Refuse to let anything stand in your way. Choose to medicate your mind by choosing to create a merry spirit on purpose.

Tell your lying-down-low-energy-lion to move over. Your tenacious tiger is the new king of the jungle!

## AND BEHOLD, THERE WAS ENERGY
## NIGHT AND DAY . . . AND EVERYONE
## COULD FEEL IT WAS GOOD!

Amazing Energy. How sweet the feeling. How great thou art.

Your tenacious tiger will love the extra zeal, zest, zing, and zip from "The Four Gospels of Gorgeous Energy!"

## BOTTOM LINE

Hello, tiger. Bye-bye, kitty. You can keep "bouncing and bouncing and bouncing" by choosing to eat, drink, sleep, and be merry.

Let's finish boot camp with a report card on your achievements:

| OLD MORNING | NEW MORNING |
|---|---|
| Six hours of sleep | Eight hours of restful sleep |
| Dull, gray room | Uplifting sunshine beaming in |
| Sugary breakfast energy bubble followed by sugar crash (or no breakfast at all) | Delicious, protein-packed, low-glycemic Revival shake with sustained energy rise |
| Watching depressing news on TV | Inspired by two-minute daily diet devotion |
| Motionless and stuffy | Brisk five-minute walk in fresh air |
| Boring same old shower | Zesty shower with music beating and stimulating candle burning |
| Rusty joints, unprotected face, and dry skin | Stretching with body moisturizing cream, SPF 20+, and beauty vitamins |
| Headed out to car mildly dehydrated | Ice-cold bottled water in hand |
| Mildewed, old food smell in car | Zipping along with lemon scent |
| Hum of traffic and monotone news on radio | Telling Diet Buddy joke on cell phone followed by more high-powered music |

| | |
|---|---|
| Trying to wake your mind up at desk | Sipping coffee or tea, alert and smiling, ready to tackle your task at hand |
| Mid-morning energy slump | Still pumping after Revival protein-packed chips and iced-cold water snack |
| **GRADE: F** *Note: Hating Life* | **GRADE: A+** ☺ *Note: Loving Life!* |

*Are you feeling it?*

Now tell me which report card do you want to take home for your mother to sign off on? Yes, I thought so.

Need to save time? Drink your shake while reading your daily diet devotion and putting your body moisturizer on. Grab a bar as you head out the door for a brisk pre-shower walk. You don't need to be a nuclear physicist to figure it out, but spending a little bit of time to get organized is important for making this easy every morning.

Will you make a commitment right now that for the next thirty days you will start your day with an energizing A+ morning? Listen to someone who took the first step:

*I made a promise to myself that I would faithfully try Revival for thirty days. I feel great. My energy level has increased and my skin appearance and hair have improved. Because of Revival, I have enough energy to do my walking and weight-bearing exercise. I eat healthier now, too! I really feel that this is the plan for the second half of my life. Thank you for creating this amazing product!*

—M. A. STEVENSON, Results not typical.†

Trust me, if you make the commitment, it will change your mind forever and put some serious energy "bling-bling" in your diet boots. Own it. Have fun with it. Use it to make you and your family gorgeous inside and out. Arise and conquer for today you have energy!

I'll show you how to stay seriously motivated for the next thirty days with *Your Daily Diet Devotions* in the next chapter. You can stay passionate about your purpose with the right daily inspiration.

## MOM'S BRIGHT BITE

You know how it is girls: You are so tired from work you can hardly undress. You kick off your shoes in random directions. You throw your clothes down instead of hanging them up like your normal neat self. And, then you make a beeline for the couch and flop down with a sigh as you close your eyes for a moment.

Then the phone rings. You listen in disbelief as your best friend starts emphatically raving about a special one-time sale going on only until 11:00 p.m. at your favorite store. Uh-oh.

A rush of adrenaline surges through your tired body, causing a strange feeling of energy to surge through your veins! You leap up, dress, and run out the door with credit card in hand to indulge in shopping satisfaction (all to the amazement of your spouse).

You literally summon up the energy from within to shop until you drop. Just goes to show us that our minds can control our energy levels by choosing to be intensely interested. I'm intensely interested in me and my family living a long and healthy life that we love. By focusing my energy on making it happen, it does. And that gives me more energy to keep making it better. So be of good cheer, and you can make it happen, too, for you and your loved ones.

## CHAPTER 7

# Your Daily Diet Devotions: Just Lose It

Remember when your mom had to wake you up for school every morning? I would have missed the school bus every day without my mom. Her daily reminder to wake up and get a move on was vital to my education.

Some things just don't change much even as adults. We could all use daily reminders from time to time to "wake up our weight loss" and educate us with slimmer habits. This chapter's purpose is to help us all stay more devoted to our diets.

In case you don't have your dictionary on hand, *devotion* means "commitment to some purpose." Are you committed to achieving a life you love? Have you purposed in your heart to become a slimmer and sexier new you?

*The new you won't happen by accident, it has to happen on purpose. Finding daily inspiration to stay passionate about our "slim and beautiful" purpose will seal the nutritional war victory. We can either choose purpose or remain porky.*

So, along with your daily fruit and vegetable servings, mom and I are going to give you several inspiring servings of hand-picked Revival goodness—from real, unpaid Revival customers, our Revival-LITES.

Every day for your first month on the *Revival Slim and Beautiful Diet* plan, mom and I will "wake you up" and help you get on the morning bus headed out of Bigville. A devotion a day will keep the doughnuts away. That's right, we are asking you to commit to thirty days of daily diet devotions, because we know it will help you develop a super-healthy habit.

Do we have a deal? How does a one-way bus ticket headed out of Bigville sound every morning? It will take less than two minutes of your time. If you miss a day, you can pick right back up where you left off.

To make each lesson sink in, we want you to circle a phrase from one of the testimonies that you find inspiring. Maybe it's about reducing your snacking and cravings, or enjoying shinier hair with smoother-looking skin. Choose something that you want to achieve. Whatever it is, dwell on it and repeat it in your mind throughout the day as you visualize your perfect new slim and beautiful body living a life it loves. We've also left you space to write down your positive thought or goal for the day corresponding to your circled phrase. Make it your daily action plan for walking further down the hill.

*Get off the sidelines and participate with us.*

## MOM'S BRIGHT BITE

### Dieter's 23-Pound Psalm

Strict is my diet. I must not want.

It maketh me to lie down at night hungry.

It leadeth me past the confectioners. It trieth my willpower.

It leadeth me in the paths of alteration for my figure's sake.

Yea, though I walk through the aisles of the pastry department,

I will buy no sweet rolls for they are fattening.

The cakes and the pies, they tempt me.

Before me is a table set with green beans and lettuce.

I filleth my stomach with liquids. My day's calorie quota runneth over.

Surely calorie and weight charts will follow me all the days of my life,

*Unless I choose not to dwell in the fear of scales forever.*

—ANONYMOUS (ADAPTED)

To download a FREE electronic copy of the devotions found here, or to get additional new devotions by e-mail that extend beyond the thirty days, visit **www.RevivalDiet.com/Resources**. You can even sign up for a free daily e-mail reminder to help you "wake up" and do your devotion.

By the way, mom and I would love to hear your success story—large or small (hopefully "smaller," right?) If you complete the thirty daily diet devotions, please let us know so we can celebrate with you! Hearing from you inspires us and makes our hard work worthwhile. It is our *fuel*, so when you become a slim and beautiful Revival-LITE, tell us your story at **www.RevivalDiet.com/Success**. Or contact us by e-mail at **Mom@Revival Diet.com** and **Doc@RevivalDiet.com**. We would love to see before and after pictures of your nutritional makeover.

We encourage you to take a sneak peak at the devotions. Thousands of people are already loving their new bodies and lives, and you will too!

## MOM'S SUGGESTION

Buy a new dress or pair of pants in the size you want to be, and then use the tag as your bookmark for your devotions.

## BEFORE WE BEGIN . . .

Mom and I would love to give a very special thanks to the thousands of Revival customers that have taken the thoughtful time to send us their success stories, so thanks! It is truly humbling to serve you.

†You can achieve wonderful typical results based on the results of Revival clinical trials. Please remember that the remarkable testimonials shared with you in this book (e.g., a loss of 20 pounds within just a few weeks; dramatic weight drops of 30 to 100 pounds or more; near-total alleviation of PMS or menopausal discomforts; or near-perfect reversal of the visible signs of

aging) are not typical results, but are included to motivate and inspire you to achieve your dreams!

Average weight loss for the Revival diet study participants was between 26 to 29 pounds in just sixteen weeks. Remember that, on any diet, nutrition or supplement plan, individual results will vary. Your weight loss results will vary based on your starting weight, activity level, and other factors. You need to faithfully follow the restricted-calorie diet plan, regular physical activity plan, and dietary supplement regimens presented in this book if you hope to achieve great weight loss, beauty, and health results documented in numerous Revival studies and other clinical trials. Typical results you can expect are discussed for each Revival study in this book. See the *Introduction* for full details. These statements have not been evaluated by the FDA. Revival products are not intended to diagnose, treat, cure, or prevent any disease.

Please contact our nutrition staff at **Nutrition@RevivalDiet.com** or **1-800-REVIVAL (1-800-738-4825)** if you have questions.

*Let's get started!*

## DAILY DIET DEVOTION #1

___ Check when completed. Circle one inspiring phrase!

*The appearance of my hair and skin has improved greatly on Revival! Shiny hair and moister, softer skin.*

—C. GILMER, Results not typical.[†]

*To date I have lost 35 pounds. I started using Revival five months ago, along with a healthy diet and exercise program. This has been an answer to my prayer! I still have about 25 pounds more to go, but now I know I will get there!*

—D. MUGERDITCHAN, Results not typical.[†]

*Having weight loss surgery has made consuming protein a top priority for me. I have tried many brands but Revival soy is not gritty and not too thick. It tastes like a chocolate milkshake—not at all like it is good for me! I need to consume 40 to 60 grams of protein daily to slow down hair loss due to protein deficiency because of the weight loss surgery. This is the easiest way for me! Thanks Revival Soy!*

—S. LODGE, Results not typical.[†]

___ I will put my diet boots on today by walking and/or staying active!

**Thoughts for today:**

### MOM'S BRIGHT BITE

Yes, my body is a temple, but I got rid of all the "ample parking in the back" with the *Revival Slim and Beautiful Diet*. You can "remodel" too!

## DAILY DIET DEVOTION #2

\_\_\_ Check when completed. Circle one inspiring phrase!

*Before Revival, I weighed 225 pounds. I had horrible night sweats and unbearable mood swings. Now, I am 80 pounds lighter and I feel great! There is not enough paper on which to tell my Revival Success Story.*

—D. HILTON, Results not typical.[†]

*With Revival, I have more energy and a positive outlook on life. My hair, skin, and nails look better. I have less sugar cravings and have more energy when I exercise. I have lost 100 pounds and need to lose 40 more. I believe that Revival can help me reach my goal weight.*

—N. HUNTER, Results not typical.[†]

*Revival was the answer to my prayers. I feel so much more alive. My hair looks great, my nails look good, and my emotions have stopped the roller coaster. I really feel great.*

—S. HAUTALA, Results not typical.[†]

\_\_\_ I will put my diet boots on today by walking and/or staying active!

## Thoughts for today:

### MOM'S BRIGHT BITE

If you have a problem exercising, try walking early in the morning before your brain figures out what it is doing—it works for me!

## DAILY DIET DEVOTION #3

\_\_\_ Check when completed. Circle one inspiring phrase!

*With Revival, I have gone from a size 14 to a size 8. I have dropped 20 pounds. and like the results. I feel better about myself and look good, too! With your product, eating healthy and exercise, it just fits! My cholesterol health is more normal too.*

—D. PENVOSE, Results not typical.[†]

*No diet program or anything else I have tried has ever been successful in helping me to lose weight. I researched Revival and took the information to my physician, who told me I could try it. I have lost 96 pounds. I started an exercise program. I still have at least another 100 pounds to lose, but I am thankful for the difference Revival has made in my life. I feel better than I have in years and finally believe there is something I can do to regain my life. Thank you.*

—L. MAYHEW, Results not typical.[†]

\_\_\_ I will put my diet boots on today by walking and/or staying active!

**Thoughts for today:**

### MOM'S BRIGHT BITE

Think about it – spending all of your money on overeating food only leaves your kids a smaller, earlier inheritance with a bigger casket bill. Do something to change it for them!

## DAILY DIET DEVOTION #4

___ Check when completed. Circle one inspiring phrase!

*The use of Revival has helped me lose more than 40 pounds, and my fifteen-year-old daughter has lost more than 15 pounds. The snack bars taste good, and they're very easy to put into the kids' backpacks for a snack before or after school sports.*

—G. WEBBER, Results not typical.[†]

*About two weeks ago I was totally upset. I got on the scales and weighed 123 pounds. I started Revival and now I'm 117 and going down. Revival has improved my well-being so much. I even feel younger, and its odd but my skin has a new glow. I'm not always thinking about food anymore. I was an evening eater. I ate most of my food after work and around bedtime. Now I'm not hungry at all, and I exercise all the time because I have this great energy I never had before I tried Revival. Thank you, Revival. You've changed my Life!*

—C. CRAWFORD, Results not typical.[†]

___ I will put my diet boots on today by walking and/or staying active!

**Thoughts for today:**

---

### MOM'S BRIGHT BITE

I repeat myself when I am hungry. I repeat myself when I am hungry.
   Stop the "diet babbling" and feel fuller by increasing your protein intake with Revival!

## DAILY DIET DEVOTION #5

___ Check when completed. Circle one inspiring phrase!

*When I first started drinking Revival, my doctor was amazed and delighted that I was able to start promoting normal cholesterol health in six weeks by drinking Revival and watching my diet. I'm not where I want to be with my diet, etc., but I am encouraged that I can get where I want to be, and I know that Revival is helping me.*

—A. STUART STONE, Results not typical.[†]

*Revival has reduced my hot flashes by about 90 percent. Revival has helped me to satisfy my chocolate cravings.*

—A.M. DENHUP, Results not typical.[†]

___ I will put my diet boots on today by walking and/or staying active!

**Thoughts for today:**

### MOM'S BRIGHT BITE

It's a great idea to pray for some serious help from above, but here's a little lighter version of *The Dieter's Prayer*:

As I wake up from my sleep, I pray my diet I may keep.
But if temptation makes me slip, I pray to God my pants won't rip!
If we continue to overeat, we will not only rip our pants, but R.I.P
as well. —ANONYMOUS

## DAILY DIET DEVOTION #6

___ Check when completed. Circle one inspiring phrase!

*I've began taking Revival and my nails look nice, my hair is growing, and I get compliments on my skin. At fifty-seven years young, I'll take all I can get. Keep up the good work. I will continue to tell everyone I meet and know.*

—V. FOSON, Results not typical.[†]

*When I first started taking Revival, I really didn't believe it would help me since I have tried so many other products. Well, the first week I started using Revival, I started sleeping through the night. Next, my nails started getting stronger and my skin became less dry. After six weeks, I had an overall sense of feeling better. I've lost 16 pounds in five weeks! I have always been completely addicted to sweets, especially gooey desserts, cakes, ice cream, etc. Now, I don't have that feeling of craving sweets any longer. Revival is truly a God-send for me. All through my life I have tried lots of diet plans, but Revival is so easy. Thank you, Dr. Tabor, for creating this amazing product that really tastes good!*

—C. NELSON, Results not typical.[†]

___ I will put my diet boots on today by walking and/or staying active!

**Thoughts for today:**

### MOM'S BRIGHT BITE

The next time someone brings you an unexpected pie or cake, try hitting him with it instead of hitting your health with it.

## DAILY DIET DEVOTION #7

___ Check when completed. Circle one inspiring phrase!

*Since having my son 5 ½ years ago, shedding the weight hasn't been easy. After having my daughter a year ago, I find myself snacking way too much. I justify it by, "Well, I have to eat something and this is all I have time for." How untrue. The first week using Revival, I lost 5 pounds! That's impressive enough for me to stick with it. I went out for brunch with a friend and I was unable to finish what I ordered, which made me feel even better. I feel more focused in other things I should be doing instead of eating.*

—J. BUGBEE, Results not typical.[†]

*After using Revival, I noticed my menstrual discomfort was greatly reduced! An added bonus was that my nails and hair grew stronger. I enjoy the health benefits associated with a doctor-approved weight management system. All thanks to Revival.*

—R. VARGAS, Results not typical.[†]

___ I will put my diet boots on today by walking and/or staying active!

**Thoughts for today:**

### MOM'S BRIGHT BITE

Think about it—the fat epidemic is widespread. Don't become a statistic!

## DAILY DIET DEVOTION #8

\_\_\_ Check when completed. Circle one inspiring phrase!

*I have lost 5 pounds, have no craving for sugar, and a lot more energy. I hope this lasts forever.*

—L. WEAVER, Results not typical.[†]

*When I use Revival daily, I feel better and have more energy. I have seen a positive difference in my hair and nails. My husband and family have noticed an improvement in my skin. (Yea! Anything to look younger!) I have not changed anything in my skin treatment regime; the soy has to be the reason for the difference. Revival tastes good and is a "no guilt" pleasure that I have faith will be beneficial to my health.*

—M. JACKSON, Results not typical.[†]

*It is much easier to maintain an appropriate weight now. My skin, nail, and hair appearance have improved so much. I feel great! People who haven't seen me for a while comment on how healthy I look, and I have recommended Revival to many friends.*

—M. FLEMING, Results not typical.[†]

\_\_\_ I will put my diet boots on today by walking and/or staying active!

## Thoughts for today:

### MOM'S BRIGHT BITE

Always laugh at yourself or you will miss 90 percent of life's fun!

## DAILY DIET DEVOTION #9

___ Check when completed. Circle one inspiring phrase!

*I've been having hot flashes and night sweats for the past two and one-half years. I thought I'd give Revival a try. The first month was wonderful—I had fewer discomforts, and it even helped me to lose 7 pounds. What a wonderful product! I've told three friends about it, and they just love your product, too. Thanks so much.*

—T. HARRIG, Results not typical.[†]

*I have always struggled with my weight, cravings, and low energy. Since menopause these things have gotten worse. Since taking Revival I have lost weight. My energy levels are increased and cravings lessened. I have fingernails again! I could not be without Revival. Revival is great tasting and easy to digest. It also has the highest amount of isoflavones [soy antioxidants] than any other product. I will never be without Revival.*

—C. JESTER, Results not typical.[†]

___ I will put my diet boots on today by walking and/or staying active!

**Thoughts for today:**

---

### MOM'S BRIGHT BITE

Be bold today—jump on your bed.

---

## DAILY DIET DEVOTION #10

___ Check when completed. Circle one inspiring phrase!

*The most immediate, dramatic difference I noticed was in my skin's appearance. At fifty-three years old, I thought my skin was beginning to look sort of dried out. After starting Revival, I noticed a big improvement, and it was not one I had even expected. I really like taking it! It tastes good and you know you are eating something healthy.*

—B. WHITE, Results not typical.[†]

*I have informed five of my friends and family members of your "Miracle Diet." I have lost 8 extra pounds that I wanted to lose in a short time. It works.*

—P. STAPLES, Results not typical.[†]

*In several weeks I have lost 9 pounds. Revival is very satisfying. I look forward to it each day.*

—A. DOMINO, Results not typical.[†]

___ I will put my diet boots on today by walking and/or staying active!

**Thoughts for today:**

### MOM'S BRIGHT BITE

Wow! Today is a new day . . . yesterday is gone along with several ounces. It feels good to be a loser.

## DAILY DIET DEVOTION #11

___ Check when completed. Circle one inspiring phrase!

*Revival has a delicious taste. I have lost 15 pounds. I had already been eating a healthy diet, exercising and losing weight, but I had "plateaued" and wasn't losing much anymore. Then I read about your product in a magazine and decided to try it. I started losing weight again. I've recommended your products to everyone I know. I love the bars! Thank you so much for your wonderful product.*

—C. SMITH, Results not typical.[†]

*A friend of mine who is a physician told me about Revival and gave me a sample. I enjoyed it right away for taste. I no longer have as many PMS discomforts. My skin has a healthy glow now, and I have more energy. I am also losing weight. I was your typical junk food junkie. I craved it and it alone. Now I crave Revival and healthy food. Praise be to God. And thank you for making this product. It is helping to turn my life around.*

—CATHY T., Results not typical.[†]

___ I will put my diet boots on today by walking and/or staying active!

**Thoughts for today:**

---

### MOM'S BRIGHT BITE

Have you been slapped with a ticket for "exceeding the *feed limit*"? Slow down your eating!

---

## DAILY DIET DEVOTION #12

___ Check when completed. Circle one inspiring phrase!

*I can see the difference in my hair, skin, and nails.*

—P. KOACH, Results not typical.[†]

*I started Revival last year and have lost 60 pounds. I have about 40 more to go and feel it will come off very easily having my Revival in the morning to get my day started right. I have tried several other brands but Revival is by far the best out there. We have also started on your multivitamin and calcium pills. Thank you for your wonderful product.*

—C. HOLTON, Results not typical.[†]

*My registered dietician recommended Revival. The results are amazing. I've lost 8 pounds; I don't crave food between breakfast and lunch and I have more energy. I've begun to exercise again. My husband can say the very same thing. It's the first diet change we've made together and that feels good, too!*

—G. BROWN, Results not typical.[†]

___ I will put my diet boots on today by walking and/or staying active!

**Thoughts for today:**

### MOM'S BRIGHT BITE

If you want something done right, do it yourself and do it for life.

## DAILY DIET DEVOTION #13

___ Check when completed. Circle one inspiring phrase!

*This is only my second week on Revival bars and I have had a huge boost in my energy level. It's amazing! The bars really do taste good and fill me up. My mood has been better (so says my boyfriend). Thanks a lot.*

—C. DODD, Results not typical.[†]

*When I first started taking Revival, I really didn't believe it would help me, since I have tried so many other products and read information that never seems to come true for me. Well, after the first week of use, I started sleeping through the night, which I have not been able to do for a long time. Over time, my nails started getting stronger, my skin became less dry, and I lost 16 pounds.*

—CAROL N., Results not typical.[†]

___ I will put my diet boots on today by walking and/or staying active!

**Thoughts for today:**

### MOM'S BRIGHT BITE

Did you know that five out of every four people have problems with fractions? Don't be made fun of because you don't examine "the math" on nutrition labels. It's easy to see how many calories and fat you are eating.

## DAILY DIET DEVOTION #14

___ Check when completed. Circle one inspiring phrase!

*After two weeks, I've noticed a 7-pound weight loss. Friends later noticed my hair was improved. I am perimenopausal, but this month I had a normal cycle for the first time in months. Thank you for a great product. There is no way I would consider going a day without Revival.*

—L. HOOVER, Results not typical.[†]

*I have lost 9 pounds since starting this program. I love the taste and feel satisfied.*

—L.A. MANSELL, Results not typical.[†]

*I saw Dr. Tabor on television talking about Revival and its health benefits. I decided to order some and give it a try. I have lost 22 pounds.*

—S. THEOBALD, Results not typical.[†]

___ I will put my diet boots on today by walking and/or staying active!

**Thoughts for today:**

---

### MOM'S BRIGHT BITE

Develop a double personality to double your results. Just repeat this fifty times:

Roses are red; Violets are blue.
I'm losing weight; And I am too!

## DAILY DIET DEVOTION #15

___ Check when completed. Circle one inspiring phrase!

*When I started Revival, I weighed in at 210 pounds. I am now 185 pounds and dropping. I am so impressed with how easy this has been—like no other time in my life before. My energy is better, and I sleep better at night. I also have less of the menopausal discomforts. This is an absolute miracle. Life is so good. Thank you, Revival.*

—G. AND J. LIND, Results not typical.[†]

*I have been using Revival for approximately three and a half months and in conjunction with a change to my diet, started walking one mile four times a week. My weight has decreased from 170 to 145 (35 pounds). I feel much better physically, and at eighty years old that is an accomplishment.*

—B. FLAGLE, Results not typical.[†]

*I'm sleeping soundly and I've lost 5 pounds! Both the Revival shakes and bars taste great! It leaves me very satisfied! Thank you!*

—J. BALLAY, Results not typical.[†]

___ I will put my diet boots on today by walking and/or staying active!

**Thoughts for today:**

### MOM'S BRIGHT BITE

Worshipping food only widens your waistline.

## DAILY DIET DEVOTION #16

___ Check when completed. Circle one inspiring phrase!

*I use Revival in the morning and it helps my hunger all day long. An added benefit is that it controls my weight and my hot flashes! Fantastic!*

—D. CAMPING, Results not typical.[†]

*I have been using your product for four months and have been amazed with the changes I've seen. My strong nails have become virtually indestructible. My hair is so soft, has a beautiful shine and is growing much faster. And a close family friend recently asked me, "What do you have all over your skin? You're glowing!" My answer, "Nothing, it's just my soy!"*

*I have noticed a significant improvement in my energy level, too. As a working mom with two small boys, I really need that. I have also noticed very positive changes in my menstrual cycle. As an educator, I love having a product that I can recommend to family, friends, colleagues and clients with 100 percent confidence. Thanks for making such a simple and highly effective product available!*

—D. GORDON, RN, Results not typical.[†]

___ I will put my diet boots on today by walking and/or staying active!

**Thoughts for today:**

### MOM'S BRIGHT BITE

Always wearing stretchy pants can be dangerous—you can't feel the growing without your "early warning" fabric in place.

## DAILY DIET DEVOTION #17

___ Check when completed. Circle one inspiring phrase!

*Revival has made me feel better, look better, and obviously get better from the inside out. Thank you so much for a wonderful product and a well run, friendly company. You have a lifelong customer in me, and I tell everyone I know.*

—P. L. KINNEY, Results not typical.[†]

*I just wanted to thank you for your great products. I'm convinced that Revival has been instrumental in helping me lose more than 50 pounds in the past six months. I exercise at least thirty minutes daily, five days a week. I'm a true believer now. I'm forty-five years old and never ever believed I could lose weight this easily—as long as I'm eating Revival, the weight is coming off like it did fifteen years ago. Thank you for producing such a great product!*

—P. HARTNETT, Results not typical.[†]

___ I will put my diet boots on today by walking and/or staying active!

**Thoughts for today:**

### MOM'S BRIGHT BITE

"To diet is to 'no' thyself," but you should never have to say no to great taste. The *Revival Slim and Beautiful Diet* is "de-lish and nutrish."

## DAILY DIET DEVOTION #18

___ Check when completed. Circle one inspiring phrase!

*I'm evangelistic about Revival. Lots of people tote water bottles everywhere, but I tote my Revival cup. When folks ask me what I'm drinking, I respond, "A chocolate shake that makes me feel great!" And then I add with a smile, "Especially during this particular stage in my life" (I'm forty-seven). Within ten minutes of drinking my daily Revival shake, I feel energetic and ready to tackle the rest of the day, as though my body has everything it needs to run at its peak performance. I've experienced a decrease in my hot flashes and a terrific method for working toward my weight-loss goals. And in the overall picture of my life, I know I'm doing something good for my body. Since I'm the forty-seven-year old mother of a vivacious seven-year-old girl, I want to insure that I stay in tip-top shape for years to come. Thank you, Revival. May your tribe increase. Be assured that I will continue to serve as a traveling evangelist for you.*

—G. IRELAND, Results not typical.[†]

___ I will put my diet boots on today by walking and/or staying active!

**Thoughts for today:**

---

### MOM'S BRIGHT BITE

A beautiful sunset, a good night's rest, and thin thighs . . . ah life CAN be good again. Persistence pays off.

## DAILY DIET DEVOTION #19

___ Check when completed. Circle one inspiring phrase!

*I want to tell you how pleased I am that I've had such great results with weight loss because of Revival. I have lost 30 pounds in four months and am certainly not starving myself at all. Thank you very much.*

—J. TRIPI, Results not typical.[†]

*I love Revival! Revival helps with my hair and my nails. Most important, it helps with my PMS and mood swings. I have tried all kinds of soy products and herb pills. Nothing else out there works like Revival. It is the best. Thank you, Revival.*

—L. BURKS, Results not typical.[†]

*I've been feeling better since I started Revival each day. I am finally feeling good enough to exercise.*

—B. WHITTER, Results not typical.[†]

___ I will put my diet boots on today by walking and/or staying active!

**Thoughts for today:**

---

### MOM'S BRIGHT BITE

"I'm not fat, I'm fluffy!" Cats are fluffy—humans are gelatinous. If you really want to be fluffy, eat cat food.

## DAILY DIET DEVOTION #20

___ Check when completed. Circle one inspiring phrase!

*I found Revival so filling that I need less food. Aside from the health benefits my husband and I derive from drinking a Revival shake each day, we find that it helps us to maintain our weight more easily. The protein is very satisfying. Our cholesterol health is more normal and we find that we have more energy. We are both in our sixties.*

—E. OKUN, Results not typical.†

*My sister-in-law is a practicing physician and provided me with information on Revival. After some research and reading, I decided to give it a try. I have lost 35 pounds and kept it off for one and a half years. I am truly thankful to have found a pleasant-tasting product that has provided me with so many health benefits. Thanks again.*

—B. RICHARD, Results not typical.†

___ I will put my diet boots on today by walking and/or staying active!

**Thoughts for today:**

### MOM'S BRIGHT BITE

Whoever said, "Dieting: It's hard by the yard, but a cinch by the inch" was right! Small, easy steps down the hill add up to big results over time.

## DAILY DIET DEVOTION #21

___ Check when completed. Circle one inspiring phrase!

*Since I have started Revival about four months ago, I have lost 30 pounds. I feel much better and I have more energy. Thank you.*

—R. ALBRANT, Results not typical.[†]

*My hair and nails are growing, which they haven't done very well before now. I love how Revival fills you up and makes you feel good.*

—W. ROSIER, Results not typical.[†]

*During perimenopause, my skin became dry and flaky. After taking Revival, I feel much better. It has definitely improved my physical well-being.*

—T. WATSON, Results not typical.[†]

___ I will put my diet boots on today by walking and/or staying active!

**Thoughts for today:**

---

### MOM'S BRIGHT BITE

I couldn't resist a few more veggie jokes:

Q: Why did the tomato go out with a prune?
A: Because he couldn't find a cute date.

## DAILY DIET DEVOTION #22

___ Check when completed. Circle one inspiring phrase!

*I sleep better than ever before. I look great! I'm forty-seven and look much younger, and now my skin and hair seem to glow. I did lose about 5 pounds. It seems like my memory is better. I have told every one I could about Revival. I am a big skeptic about anything and everything, so this came as a big surprise. I am religious about Revival. I feel it has saved my life, sanity, health, and marriage.*

—L. SARGEANT, Results not typical.[†]

*I was trying to get through menopause with a good diet, exercise, and with a few herbs. I still had multiple hot flashes, a few night sweats, trouble sleeping, and some decrease in hair health. Revival has been wonderful! After three months all my discomforts were much improved. I ran out of product for six days and the discomforts started to return. It's a great, quick breakfast (I add a small banana and ice cubes for a thick shake), and I don't get hungry until lunchtime. Thanks.*

—P. MCSWEENEY, Results not typical.[†]

___ I will put my diet boots on today by walking and/or staying active!

## Thoughts for today:

### MOM'S BRIGHT BITE

I used to think the middle age spread was just a myth. Life's truths can be so crushing without proper preparation.

## DAILY DIET DEVOTION #23

___ Check when completed. Circle one inspiring phrase!

*Revival has helped me lose 15 pounds. This extra weight made me discouraged. I feel much better now. Thanks, Revival! Revival has also allowed my PMS to be bearable. Revival allowed me to feel better about myself and helps me sleep like a baby. I am healthy and I feel great. Once again, thank you!*

—A. TASK, Results not typical.[†]

*I decided to make some lifestyle changes in an attempt to improve my health. I weighed 234 pounds (at five-foot-five). I started eating a more healthy diet, cut back on portions, and started walking a little everyday. I also ordered Revival. I now weigh 130 pounds (a 104-pound weight loss). I'm very pleased with how I look and feel now; I get so many compliments it is embarrassing. Thank you for a wonderful product.*

—D. HUNTER, Results not typical.[†]

___ I will put my diet boots on today by walking and/or staying active!

**Thoughts for today:**

### MOM'S BRIGHT BITE

Q: What vegetable did Noah leave OFF the Ark?

A: Leeks.

## DAILY DIET DEVOTION #24

___ Check when completed. Circle one inspiring phrase!

*My energy is up, skin clearer, less cramping, and fewer mood swings with PMS. In general, I just feel so much better. Revival is very filling with great taste.*

—M. MICALLEF, Results not typical.[†]

*I feel mentally changed. My weight is gradually dropping off, and my appetite and sugar cravings are drastically reduced (a major plus). I also have an overall sense of balance and well-being.*

—D. SOLOMON, Results not typical.[†]

*I am fifty-two years old and have tried everything for my weight. So, I tried Revival for a week and can see the difference already. I've lost 5 pounds by eating less and eating Revival. I feel great! I have cut down on my food, and have noticed that I am not as hungry all the time.*

—G. REISS, Results not typical.[†]

___ I will put my diet boots on today by walking and/or staying active!

**Thoughts for today:**

### MOM'S BRIGHT BITE

Getting "fed up" with goodies only leads to becoming "fed up" with your body.

## DAILY DIET DEVOTION #25

___ Check when completed. Circle one inspiring phrase!

*Revival has helped me in a lot of ways: 1) I feel healthier—my skin, hair, and nails are healthier, and 2) my body fat has reduced. Thanks for caring.*

—M. GAINEY, Results not typical.[†]

*I just started on Revival and lost 2 pounds the first week. I really only lose weight when I starve myself, but didn't have to do that with Revival. My cravings for sweets are much better.*

—B. BOWERS, Results not typical.[†]

*I am in perimenopause and have been experiencing night sweats on a regular basis. Within two weeks of starting Revival, my night sweats decreased substantially. I also lost 3 pounds after the first week of using Revival daily.*

—J. STRONG, Results not typical.[†]

___ I will put my diet boots on today by walking and/or staying active!

**Thoughts for today:**

---

### MOM'S BRIGHT BITE

Q: What did the lettuce say to the celery?
A: Quit stalking me!

Celery filled with organic, crunchy peanut butter makes a great snack to stalk Mrs. Thin.

## DAILY DIET DEVOTION #26

___ Check when completed. Circle one inspiring phrase!

*Revival has helped slow down the hot flashes, and helped my hair and nails. I now sleep well.*

—B. MILLER, Results not typical.[†]

*After using Revival for two months, I noticed my appetite decreased. Not only am I losing some extra weight, I also have more energy and a better outlook. I'm glad I stuck with it! I plan to stay on Revival for a long time.*

—C. HETZELL, Results not typical.[†]

*Revival has given me a convenient way to get the daily protein my body requires, and in a super tasty way! I recently had gastric bypass surgery. Losing 123 pounds in eight months can have some serious side effects without the proper nutrition. Revival brought me the proper nutrition at a great price. I can't wait to tell all my friends. I have already posted all the information on our support group home page. Thanks for a great product!*

—M. KRAFT, Results not typical.[†]

___ I will put my diet boots on today by walking and/or staying active!

**Thoughts for today:**

---

### MOM'S BRIGHT BITE

Nothing feels as good as fitting in pants that didn't fit last week! Feel it, and do it.

---

## DAILY DIET DEVOTION #27

___ Check when completed. Circle one inspiring phrase!

*I haven't been on Revival long but I can tell I have more energy already. My hot flashes are better. My woozy feelings are almost gone. I have Revival at lunch. I've lost 5 to 6 pounds already. I don't get hungry.*

—C. GAMBILL, Results not typical.[†]

*I was so tired of feeling tired all the time. I could hardly function at work. During menopause, my weight started climbing. When I heard about Revival and how Dr. Tabor's mother seemed to have similar discomforts, I decided to give it a try. I was pleasantly surprised at how delicious Revival was. Almost immediately, approximately three days, I felt better. My discomforts started to lessen. My husband and friends noticed I was happier and had more energy. Everyone wanted to know what I was doing, and I was very happy to share the good news. The bonus is I am losing weight. I just want everyone to feel as good as I do! Thank you, Dr. Tabor and everyone at Revival, for giving me my life back.*

—K. MENTZ, Results not typical.[†]

___ I will put my diet boots on today by walking and/or staying active!

**Thoughts for today:**

### MOM'S BRIGHT BITE

Choose to use your lips for good! Try more kissing and less "dishing."

## DAILY DIET DEVOTION #28

___ Check when completed. Circle one inspiring phrase!

*The Revival shakes are wonderful for weight control. I drink one in the morning and I'm full until lunch at 1:30 or 2:00. I have lost 25 pounds since April by using these products with my weight-loss program. Thank you!*

—C. S. TRAVERS, Results not typical.[†]

*I am very new to the Revival family! I have been using Revival for approximately two weeks and have lost 4 pounds surprisingly. I am so psyched and enthused about this fantastic product. I am exercising (run/walk) four days a week. I have never been so happy, energetic, and impressed.*

—C. JOHNSON, Results not typical.[†]

*I've been using Revival for only about four weeks now, and I've already noticed increased energy, a 5-pound weight loss, and lessened menopausal discomforts.*

—J. MOORE, Results not typical.[†]

___ I will put my diet boots on today by walking and/or staying active!

**Thoughts for today:**

### MOM'S BRIGHT BITE

Music, music, music . . . put it on, turn it up and move around—something may fall off, including pounds!

## DAILY DIET DEVOTION #29

___ Check when completed. Circle one inspiring phrase!

*I've been on Revival now for eleven weeks and it has helped in the following ways:*

1. *I've only had one night sweat in this time. That's such a relief.*
2. *It has increased my energy.*
3. *My hair feels so much stronger and silkier (soft and shiny now).*
4. *It has helped my nails.*
5. *I've lost weight and I love it. It helped me get rid of that extra weight around my waist.*

—C. WHITE, Results not typical.[†]

*I started eating the Revival bars and in a matter of days the difference was unbelievable. Now I find I don't need that continual eating, searching for food for energy. I will never give up Revival. This is the answer my body was craving.*

—B. ZAJICEK, Results not typical.[†]

___ I will put my diet boots on today by walking and/or staying active!

**Thoughts for today:**

### MOM'S BRIGHT BITE

The big bad wolf loves the smell of bacon—let's not invite unwanted health problems to the door of our homes.

## DAILY DIET DEVOTION #30

Our thoughts for today:

Congratulations! You have made it to the thirtieth day of diet devotions. We would circle you if we could, because you inspire us!

*Take a day off and celebrate your success so far with one or more of these doctor-recommended and mom-approved suggestions:*

1. Full-body massage.
2. Manicure and facial.
3. Makeover.
4. Babysitter and shopping spree for new clothes!
5. Short drive and picnic.
6. Hot bath/shower and favorite movie with popcorn.
7. New puppy (your new walking buddy!)

Please be sure to tell us your success story at **www.RevivalDiet.com/Success**.

## CHAPTER 8

# Escape Your Hormonal Hades, the Valley of Dry Bones, and a Broken Heart: Soy Meets Girl

*The first thing I noticed with Revival use was reduction in hot flashes and night sweats. Oh, did I mention I have lost 15 pounds? I love Revival.*

—D. MARTIN, Results not typical.[†]

*I endured PMS for years. Mood swings and bloating were the worst. I can honestly say that they're all better! Amazing! I have lost 10 pounds!! My hair, skin, and nails all look improved. Thanks so much! Keep up the good work.*

—R. DAVIS, Results not typical.[†]

*Since I started consuming Revival products, I've noticed less hot flashes, better sleep, less mood swings, and I have even lost inches. Thank God for*

---

[†]Results not typical, but included to motivate you. Individual results vary. You must follow the calorie-restricted diet plan, physical activity plan, and dietary supplement regimens presented in this book if you hope to achieve great weight loss, beauty, and health results. see *Introduction* and specific studies presented in this book for typical results. These statements have not been evaluated by the Food and Drug Administration. Revival is not intended to diagnose, treat, cure, or prevent any disease.

*Revival! I enjoy restful nights, peace of mind and daily energy to enjoy life as it should be enjoyed—naturally.*

—V. A. RIVERA, Results not typical.†

"Beep! Beep!" Move over because I have *energy* on board!

Your tenacious tiger is sprinting down the open road faster than a road runner when it happens . . . your tiger stumbles over a Tasmanian devil . . . (I credit my dad for teaching me such descriptive medical terminology!)

"Rut-row!"

As you awaken, you read the large road sign above you:


## WELCOME TO HORMONAL HADES, POPULATION: 1 VERY MISERABLE WOMAN

Hormonal imbalances have ambushed you with PMS and menopause. It's a hostage crisis situation—you are trapped, and men-are-on-pause.

> **FACT:** While declining estrogen levels, menopause, and PMS are all normal parts of aging (i.e., not considered a disease), they certainly don't feel normal.

As you know by now, I created the original Revival soy product to naturally rescue my mom from a midlife meltdown that included a firestorm of menopausal hot flashes, night sweats, and hot-tempered mood swings. It would be silly for me to go into a detailed discussion of what hot flashes, PMS, or other hormonal discomforts are because: 1) you already understand exactly what they are in *excruciating* detail if you are trapped by them, 2) a man can explain a hot flash or PMS about as well as he can give birth to a baby, and 3) this book is about straight-forward natural solutions, not long definitions. Let's just suffice it to say that having your life "charbroiled" by PMS or menopause isn't exactly having life your way or loving it. I'm here to rescue you, too.

Thankfully, not only did mom survive midlife, but she has also flourished into a beautiful bouquet of roses—I'm proud of her! It's been a "Soy Meets Girl" love story ever since Revival gave her a great life back.

---

**FACT:** Thousands of other women are now living lives they love with Revival. They've not only escaped their Hormonal Hades, but they've done it in *style*.

---

It's inspiring—just listen!

*Revival products have helped with my weight loss and hot flashes. Hot flashes are nearly all gone and when I do get one, it is mild. The bars and chips help curb my appetite which has helped me lose 30 pounds. I love the variety and the taste.*

—C. TUSCHL, Results not typical.[†]

*Hello, I am a sixty-one-year-old female Revival auto-delivery member, and I have been using Revival for several months, with excellent results. My hot flashes and night sweats are so much better, my skin looks great. I sleep like a Chihuahua between his master's knees. My mind is clear and sharp with a feeling of joy and well-being.*

—P. J. WOOD, Results not typical.[†]

*Less hot flashes or night sweats, since taking Revival. I have a more stable mood which is great. My hair is improving and I have more energy.*

—M. D. SIEWERT, Results not typical.[†]

*On top of the reduction of hot flashes, I have noticed that my nails are nice and shiny. Try Revival—You'll like it!*

—J. MOESSNER, Results not typical.[†]

## CLINICALLY PROVEN
## ANTI-TASMANIAN-DEVIL BENEFITS

If you are being tormented in your own Hormonal Hades (some women call it their "year-round personal summer"), keep your cool for just a bit longer because the Tasmanian devil catcher from Animal Control is already on his way! Before I rescue you with my "C-P-R Escape Plan" (which I'll explain later in this chapter), I want to summarize a Revival menopause research study. This study was conducted at a major academic medical center known around the world, so I must warn you to be prepared for a complicated, difficult-to-understand scientific graph. Ready? Take a big breath and view carefully . . .

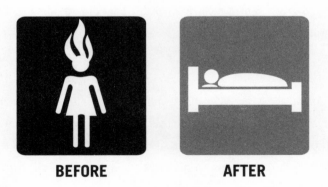

**BEFORE**           **AFTER**

If you need help understanding these results, please contact my nutrition staff *immediately!* This Revival study, conducted at one of America's best hospitals, along with more than twenty other published studies on soy protein and soy antioxidants for midlife health, verifies exactly what mom and thousands of Revival-LITES are already feeling and loving.

**FACT:** Revival Works!

Positive improvements in comfort levels of almost 40 percent were seen within three months of consuming just one naturally concentrated Revival shake (or bar) supplement with 20 grams of soy protein and 160 milligrams of soy antioxidants. The average scores in four separate medically established menopausal discomfort categories were measured. Take a peek and "feel" the results yourself:

1. *The Vasomotor category (36 percent improvement) includes:* Reduced hot flashes, night sweats, and sweating.
2. *The Psychosocial category (40 percent improvement) includes:* Reduced dissatisfaction with personal life, feeling anxious or nervous, experiencing poor memory, accomplishing less than normal, feeling moody, being impatient with other people, and wanting to be alone.
3. *The Physical category (30 percent improvement) includes:* Reduced tired feelings, difficulty sleeping, decrease in physical strength, decrease in stamina, lack of energy, dry skin, weight gain, change in appearance/texture of skin, feeling bloated, flatulence or gas pains, and frequent urination.
4. *The Sexual category (36 percent improvement) includes:* Reduced change in sexual desire, vaginal dryness during intercourse, and avoiding intimacy.

## MOM'S BRIGHT BITE

For me, Revival is like Eve's leaves—it meets a real need. I would feel "nutritionally naked" without it.

## PMS . . . PERPETUAL MUNCHING SPREE . . . PUNISH MEN SEVERLY?

When life tastes this good, the good news just keeps getting better: Revival may also lessen PMS.

For millions of women, PMS is definitely no picnic in the park. PMS is similar to having a mini-menopause each month, because after your estrogen spikes it rapidly falls. This can produce menopausal-like estrogen withdrawal discomforts, including hot flashes, bloating, and mood swings. Several human studies indicate that regular soy consumption may support better menstrual health and lessen PMS by favorably balancing estrogen levels and altering estrogen metabolism. And that's great news for women—and men—everywhere.

---

### MOM'S BRIGHT BITE

**What does PMS or menopause mean to you?**
Here are a few of my favorite PMS definitions:

- Profoundly Miserable Sleep
- Psychotic Mood Shift
- Punish Men Severely
- Pardon My Sobbing
- Puffy Mid-Section
- Pack My Stuff

- Pass My Shotgun
- Perpetual Munching Spree
- Pepperoni Mushrooms Sausage
- Pass My Sweatpants
- Pass Me Sweets

All of these really make me laugh, but the sad truth is that hormonal swings can make each of us feel like packing our stuff up (or packing it in) at times. Revival helps me to be more balanced naturally, and that's something I feel really great about deep down in my body and mind. I tell Doc that he gets an A+ from me.

---

Listen to the harmonious words Revival-LITES are shouting about PMS:

*I love Revival! Revival helps with my hair and my nails. Most important, it helps with my PMS and mood swings. I have tried all kinds of soy products and herb pills. Nothing else out there works like Revival. It is the best. Thank you, Revival.*

—L. BURKS, Results not typical.[†]

*During my PMS weeks I'm normally irritable, constantly hungry, etc., but this time it passed without notice!*

—K. E. BOUCHARD, Results not typical.[†]

*My energy is up, skin looks clearer, less cramping, and fewer mood swings with PMS. In general, I just feel so much better. Revival is very filling with great taste.*

—M. MICALLEF, Results not typical.[†]

## THE VALLEY OF DRY BONES AND A BROKEN HEART: 1 MILE AHEAD

Soy's benefits don't end with simply helping you escape your Hormonal Hades. With disappearing estrogen levels during midlife (losses can start as early as age thirty-five), you may find that your road map to health also disappears. Before you know it, you can find yourself lost in several places which we'll discuss next that are more treacherous than your Hormonal Hades!

### The Valley of Dry Bones: Don't break your beauty dreams!

The Valley of Dry Bones is one of the most dangerous and ugly places on earth, haunted with broken hips, fractured bones, and horrifying hunchbacks bent on destroying your beauty dreams.

**FACT:** Healthy facial and skeletal bones
are essential for a beautiful face and body.

Your bones are continuously remodeling through an ongoing cycle in which old bone is broken down and new bone is built. Rapidly declining estrogen levels during menopause can cause rapid bone loss because the remodeling cycle drastically changes for the worse. Bone breakdown begins happening faster than when new bone is rebuilt, and you lose more calcium through your urine. Over time, your bones become "wrinkled," weak and brittle with tiny holes inside. The osteoporosis monster has hatched, and if you ignore it, it can turn your beautiful life upside down with broken bones, hip fractures, or a sunken face. My "C-P-R Escape Plan" that I will share with you in just a moment will help you promote better bone health. Being stranded in the Valley of Dry Bones without an action plan is unwise.

### A Broken Heart: Don't let it kill your total-body beauty!

Cardiovascular disease is the number-one killer of women and men. Period.

Having a hot flash or PMS is awful, but having a life-changing (or life-ending) sudden heart attack is atrocious. Your healthy heart is vital for pumping rosy oxygen-rich blood and beautifying nutrients to every single cell of your body inside and out, so nourishing and protecting your heart should be at the very top of your priority list. Looking beautiful and healthy is impossible without a healthy heart. A severely damaged heart will diminish your beautiful face's appearance and your skin's glow.

High levels of bad cholesterol (called *LDL* cholesterol) in your bloodstream can kill your health and beauty dreams. The bad cholesterol sticks to the inside of your arteries, eventually clogging them shut with devastating plaques. Without oxygen and nutrients, your cells begin to starve and die. It isn't a pretty sight. I don't think you want to starve your cells any more than you want to starve your own children.

Ready to keep your distance from a broken heart by promoting normal cholesterol levels?

## "I'M READY TO ESCAPE, SO TELL ME THE C-P-R ESCAPE PLAN—NOW!"

Okay! Freedom awaits your sweet escape using my simple "C-P-R Escape Plan."[†] Resuscitate your health with these three easy steps:

### First Step = C: "Call" Animal Control ASAP

Call Animal Control as soon as possible at **1-800-REVIVAL** or **www.RevivalDiet.com** to chase your pesky Tasmanian devil away. In the Revival menopause study, women simply enjoyed one naturally concentrated Revival soy protein bar or shake supplement daily. It's easy to enjoy a bar or shake as part of your daily eating pattern (on either the milk-protein-based diet or soy-protein-based diet). You can also enjoy a naturally concentrated bar or shake supplement alone if you aren't actively using *The Revival Slim & Beautiful Diet* for weight loss.

You may experience a quick improvement in your energy levels and lessening in your menopausal or PMS discomforts after starting Revival. Mom experienced an immediate boost in her energy and a noticeable hot flash reduction within three days. Individual results vary, but be consistent daily over time for best results.

I believe naturally concentrated Revival soy bar and shake supplements are effective because they contain an unprecedented amount of soy antioxidants (isoflavones): equivalent to 6 cups of a typical soymilk (without the soy taste of course) *combined* with 20 grams of soy protein. We go to the heart of the soybean to harvest the naturally rich goodness without the need for chemical concentration. The protein *and* antioxidant combination likely produces a beautiful, synergistic symphony involving "all of soy's instruments" that soy pills simply can't duplicate.

Promote better bone health to start walking away from the Valley of Dry Bones. Enjoy naturally concentrated Revival soy protein, rich in soy antioxidants, combined with bone-healthy calcium, to support healthy bones (including facial bones) by replacing the lost calcium and supporting normal calcium metabolism. Enjoying Revival milk-protein-based products may help maintain better bone health, too. Choose to be a "bonehead" by eating soy protein, milk protein, and calcium daily. Don't let an unchallenged calcium deficiency break your beauty dreams into pieces. Long-term daily consumption is important for bone health support. Keep your healthcare provider involved in your escape. You may need a yearly bone scan, particularly if you are over sixty-five years old. Physical activity is also paramount to steer clear from the Valley of Dry Bones, so keep on walking!

Promote normal cholesterol levels to help avoid a "Broken Heart." Daily use of Revival is the A+ answer.

---

**FACT:** A large Revival study, funded by the National Institutes of Health (NIH), has found that 20 grams of Revival soy protein containing 160 milligrams of soy antioxidants (found in one naturally concentrated bar or shake supplement), helps to promote normal cholesterol health.

---

With so many additional studies finding that soy promotes normal cholesterol levels, the Food and Drug Administration (FDA) has issued an official government health claim that, "Diets low in saturated fat and cholesterol that include 25 grams of soy protein a day may reduce the risk of heart disease."

Eating 25 grams of soy protein per day is easy to achieve as part of your daily eating pattern. Simply choose one Revival bar or shake (regular or naturally concentrated to enjoy 20 grams of soy protein) and one Revival snack (e.g., Revival protein chips to enjoy an additional 7 grams of soy protein).

The NIH-funded study also found that regular enjoyment may promote normal "HDL-cholesterol" (the good cholesterol) health.

In the Revival Diet clinical trial, both the milk-protein-based diet and soy-protein-based diet were found to promote normal cholesterol levels, normal blood pressure, and maintenance of proper blood sugar levels.

Are you starting to get the picture? Look at this:

*I have been using Revival soy drinks and/or bars almost daily for the past four months. I am happy to report that Revival is promoting normal choles-terol health. My hot flashes have diminished. I did notice that if I left off the Revival plan for three or four days, I would start getting hot flashes again, but they stopped as soon as I got back on Revival. And I am very happy to report that I have lost 17 pounds during that time.*

—C. Van Hoozier, M.D., Results not typical.[†]

Choose to promote normal cholesterol levels. Don't leave home without a healthy heart! If you have a history of being overweight, having high cho-lesterol, or smoking, take special care of your arteries and heart now and in the future because  you may already have existing damage. I recommend that you see your healthcare provider for a complete evaluation to be on the safe side. You may need prescription medications if diet and exercise alone fail to normalize your cholesterol.

---

## MOM'S BRIGHT BITE

You may be in menopause if you need to write Post-It notes with your kids' names on them!

---

Let's see . . . where were we headed . . . oh yes, memory!
Keep in mind that several human studies indicate regular soy consumption

can also support normal memory health in both women and men. Revival may help make your short-term memory annoyances less annoying.

### Second Step = P: "Pump" in the Troops—Extra Calcium, Vitamins, and Antioxidants.

Because estrogen is a potent connective tissue stimulator in your skin, hair, nails, and bones, declining estrogen levels bode poorly for beauty. Skin looks thinner at an accelerated pace and becomes dry. Hair looks more dull and fragile. Nails appear brittle and split. Midlife can be an ugly event to watch unfold unless intervention is launched.

As discussed, menopause's other impact on your health and beauty is *accelerated* calcium loss, which can knock your bones down for the final count. It's an insidious, dirty assault that can leave you slumped over, fragile, and less than graceful.

> **FACT:** You don't have to become a martyr of midlife by letting the change of life be an unchallenged, permanent change for the worse.

New dietary supplement science can be part of your saving grace—you no longer have to just stand there and turn the other cheek as you watch your skin, hair, nails, and normal bone health "burn up" in your Hormonal Hades. If you turn the other cheek to midlife's woes, you won't have much of a cheek (or anything else) left before too long.

You can fight back by sending in the right health and beauty troops. Extra calcium (1000 to 1300 milligrams per day), vitamins, minerals, antioxidants, herbs, essential fatty acids from oils (Omega 3 and 6), peptides, and other clinically proven beauty ingredients support, maintain, and nourish every cell of your body.

Ask the search-and-rescue team at Animal Control (i.e., my expert nutrition staff) for our very latest recommended support solutions. New nutrition science emerges almost weekly, but you can rely on us to do all of hard staying-up-to-date work for you. Relax, we have it covered.

Choose to fight back and promote better health by pumping in the right perfect-and-protect troops to march alongside Revival soy-protein-based and milk-protein-based products.

### Step Three = R: Rehabilitate Your Determination to Succeed Every Day!

*Never, never, never, never give up.*
—WINSTON CHURCHILL

Reaffirm in your heart daily that you will never fail—that you will never, ever let your health or beauty be left behind by the ravages of time. You can ensure freedom by keeping your cross hairs aimed precisely every single day at the principles you have been taught in this plan:

**Picture clearly** the beautiful, healthy life you want to live and love.

**Walk** down the **Revival Slim and Beautiful Diet** path with me.

**Wield** your superhero powers for permanent weight loss with the Ten Psychological Commandments.

**Accelerate** your weight loss with the Fifteen Physical Laws.

**Flee** the Seven Deadly Skin Sins.

**Perfect and Protect** with the latest nutritional makeover beauty ingredient technologies.

**Energize** gorgeously with the Four Gospels.

**Uplift and motivate** yourself daily with the Diet Devotions.

**Help** your Diet Buddy, family, and friends achieve their dreams, too.

**Become** stronger by leading a Revival Diet Small Group as a "shrink."

Choose to never stop religiously reviewing and practicing these principles. Being in the best physical health and psychological state possible makes your escape from Hormonal Hades, the Valley of Dry Bones, and a broken heart easier. And not only will you escape, but you will do it *in style*.

## BOTTOM LINE

The three steps of my C-P-R Escape Plan work together for your good when you choose to use all of them. You will be more than a conqueror when you resuscitate yourself and live a life that you love in hormonal bliss.

---

### MOM'S BRIGHT BITE[†]

I read about the seven dwarves of menopause online: Itchy, Witchy, Sweaty, Sleepy, Bloated, Forgetful, and Psycho! It doesn't sound like these guys would help Snow White out much.

I'm so grateful that my real "Doc" showed up and helped me survive midlife! I want to share more details with you about my story, and how Revival gave me back the *control* over my life and health, because I believe it will help many of you.

Menopause affects each of us differently, but it hit me between the eyes like a sharp, unrelenting, hot ray of sun. Forget the cute red hats ladies—I was made a member of the Red *Hot* Society without even asking to join! When you are tossing and turning at night with an unending barrage of heat waves rolling over your body, a pea under your mattress sheet (or even a coconut under your mattress) wouldn't cause any discomfort compared to the power-surge attack.

Early on when my hot flashes first started, I tore the cover off a large yellow notepad and kept it in my nightstand drawer so I could fan myself *a la carte* throughout the night. It was my best friend for many years (it was ragged, torn and bent by the time I threw it out) until Doc rescued me with Revival from my personal heat wave and other midlife woes.

At times before Revival I had been known to open the freezer door to catch one second of that cool breeze wafting from the amazing box. I would frequently stagger out of bed, throw off my gown, and walk out the door in the cold winter night just to get some immediate relief. It's good thing our porch was out of our neighbor's view! My husband was delighted at first as I ripped off my gown and declared how hot I was. But his joy was short lived when I shouted, "Don't-touch-me-your-hands-are-so-hot!" and meant it.

I also kept him up all hours of the night with the covers flying this way and that way. Incessant digging in the drawer for my homemade cardboard fan and balm for my dry lips earned me the nickname of "Squirrel." Oh, there was also the nightly disturbance of my half-asleep moaning as I awoke sweating, followed by my getting out of bed to change into dry clothes.

I should say here, that I am not one to endure in silence or alone. I prefer company with my misery. So menopause didn't just affect me; my husband was kidnapped and forced to ride along on the dismal road. God help all husbands living through this now! I always wondered why there are such a large number of divorces in midlife—now I know what may contribute to them!

During this time of trying to live with the heat, I had other things going on that were uncomfortable and unsightly. First there was what I call the Great Sahara Desert Syndrome: my eyes, skin, and whole body were becoming dry. I could, and did, scratch my name on my leg just to show my husband I could do it (I think it was about 3:00 a.m. one morning).

I remember wondering how so many women deal with this horrible time of life. As I talked to other women going through the change, I heard many stories of how they were barely hanging on, despite using many various strategies. Midlife can wreck even the best of marriages.

Unlike so many of the ladies I talked with, my husband and I had always communicated like two Chatty Cathy dolls, so he knew exactly what I was going through. He was a true buddy and advocate determined to find and implement something that would help "us." Just his use of the word "us"—instead of "you"—says so much about my man. I really got the prize when I picked him some forty years ago.

I could write a more detailed, tear-jerking saga of my own life here, but I know all of you who have experienced the change of hormonal seasons could write your own saga.

*I want to give you hope.*

Perhaps it is no accident that menopause and the infamous years of midlife crisis seem to correspond. Your waistline starts expanding (rapidly). Have you heard about the furniture disease of midlife? Your chest falls to your drawers.

Your hair either turns gray or turns brittle (or both)! When you start to jog you realize that your mind is about one hundred feet ahead of your body. A simple basketball game or game of tennis puts you at risk for losing a toenail. When you lean over and look in a mirror, you imagine yourself being eighty soon (I do not recommend you ever imagine this, for obvious reasons). You walk slower when you get up out of bed to go to the bathroom during the night. Your aches and pains seem to be more noticeable in the morning.

And I saved the best for last: your skin starts visibly sagging.

The only thing I like about the term *midlife crisis* is that I'm a problem solver, so when I see a crisis, it's an invitation to find a solution. Today I can thank God for hot flashes, because they drove Doc and I to find the help I needed—help I now excitedly share with other women in need. The solution was definitely not hair color, artificial nails, facials, a new husband, or a sports car. I needed real help, starting from the inside out . . . and that is exactly what I got with Revival.

With the first Revival naturally concentrated soy shake that Aaron formulated for me, I immediately found I had more energy. Yes, increased energy and a clearer head were the very first benefits I experienced. I probably was not getting all the protein I needed, at least not the right kind of protein that was so complete with amino acids. It felt like my body soaked up the shake as a thirsty plant would soak up water. And my body responded just like a flower to a good watering.

About three days after I started drinking the "delicious wonder shake," my hot flashes began to go down in number. Until then, I had about fifty or more hot flashes a day—and that didn't include the ones that plagued my nights. I thought, at first, *Okay, this is one of those "placebo effect" things. It isn't real, and I will be digging for my fan in a few hours.* But the relief continued.

As the days turned into weeks, the hot flashes continued to subside. I could sleep all the way through the night without discomfort (or digging like a squirrel)! Around the third month on my "Revival ride," my skin, hair, and nails, started showing visible signs of real improvements, and by the sixth month it was easy to see. My hormonal moodiness was also washed away. I was happy! And my husband was even more overjoyed.

I just could not believe this was happening. My parched body actually felt as though someone had turned my natural sprinkler system back on, and it was working from the inside out. When I went for my regular yearly checkup, my doctor was amazed, and started recommending Revival to other patients.

Now, I get compliments all of the time on my dewy-looking skin and healthy-looking hair and nails. I never had particularly good skin before Revival, so to hear someone tell me this is so amazing. It helps negate the impact of midlife. An encouraging word goes a long way.

I needed energy to help me get through menopause. When Revival began helping with the hot flashes and night sweats, I could finally get a good night's sleep which helped me have even more energy.

Then my weight! I actually began slimming up instead of spreading out. Ladies and gentlemen, you do not have to be fifty and fat. No product is going to decrease your actual age, but some can make you feel and look younger. Revival did that for me, and continues to give me the energy and midlife relief I need each day to press on.

The crisis has been taken out of my midlife!

My husband, my family, and I can enjoy these years as a gift of life from our Creator and stop focusing on the negatives of growing older. In fact, my husband and I started telling our kids that, "Life begins at fifty!" We are truly kicking up our heels in midlife and looking forward to finding all the treasure in the golden years before us (yes, my husband uses Revival products every day, too).

*I have my hope back, my health back, and the feeling of control in my life.*

My sincere hope is that Doc's research, Revival, and this book can give you and your loved ones the same.

On the first page of this book, I promised you that we would fight an all-out nutritional war against ugly, gelatinous fat, low energy, appearance of wrinkles, dull hair, and weak nails to produce a "slim and beautiful" new you. Based on the Revival research results, I believe that Mom and I have given you exactly the right diet boots to make your dream of a beautiful life you love achievable.

As she and I discussed how to possibly say "goodbye" at the end of this book, we decided to tell you that we are imagining you healthy, energetic, and beautiful, enjoying good food with your good friends, clapping your hands with joy as we often do. The thought brings a smile to our faces and inspires us to work harder.

It would be great to hear from you. You can e-mail us at **Mom@RevivalDiet.com** and **Doc@RevivalDiet.com**. Please do send before and after pictures!

Stop by to see a special video message from Mom and I at **www.Revival Diet.com** and sign up for a free beauty research newsletter for your long-term motivation.

We will leave you with one last **FACT**:

**F:** Follow the downhill path to your dreams.
**A:** Act today because every day is a gift.
**C:** Contact Animal Control.
**T:** Tend to your family and friends too.

*And, today you will be in paradise!*

CHOOSE to rule your health and beauty world with the Revival Slim & Beautiful Diet Resources. Please contact us if you need help at **1-800-REVIVAL** (1-800-738-4825), **www.RevivalDiet.com**, or **Nutrition@ RevivalDiet.com**.

    A.  Become a "Shrink": Host a Revival Diet Small Group!
    B.  Revival Slim & Beautiful Diet Plan Summaries
    C.  Daily Eating Pattern Templates
    D.  Medical Study References for the Intellectually Curious
    E.  Healthcare Provider Patient Samples Program
    F.  Nutrition Staff & Order Information

## A. BECOME A "SHRINK": HOST A REVIVAL DIET SMALL GROUP!

What's the only thing better than a Diet Buddy? Diet Buddies!

*You can lead others down the hill to a more beautiful, healthier life as a Revival Diet "Shrink." Improving and saving lives will help you become stronger in your personal walk.*

### How Do I Become a Shrink? And What Is Involved in Leading a Group?

It's super simple to become a shrink and lead a Small Group. Download the free Revival Diet Small Group Guide at **www.RevivalDiet.com/Resources**, call us at **1-800-REVIVAL** (1-800-738-4825), or e-mail **Nutrition@RevivalDiet.com**.

The guide shows you step-by-step how to host a thirty-minute weekly support group meeting at your home, office, church, or social group. The meetings last for a short six weeks, but can be extended if your group sees fit. Recommended group size is six to twelve people.

Each meeting consists of a short teaching session (fifteen minutes on a key diet principle) and an accountability and group discussion session (fifteen minutes). The guide gives you the exact teaching points used for each teaching session, and it instructs you how to direct your group during each accountability and discussion session. We even include announcements that you can personalize and post to recruit Small Group members.

Your Revival Diet Small Group can up set up a free online Diet Buddy Group at **www.RevivalDiet.com/Resources** so the progress of each member can be tracked and shared online with the entire Small Group for the ultimate accountability, motivation, support, and "nutritional makeover" success.

A faith-based, non-denominational version is also available for download, which adds weekly Scripture readings and a prayer journal for participants. A video-based Small-Group curriculum will be available soon, so please contact us for the latest details.

Lead others to strengthen yourself and you will find your entire world becomes a more beautiful place!

## B. REVIVAL SLIM AND BEAUTIFUL
## DIET PLAN SUMMARIES

For your viewing pleasure and culinary convenience:

### Rapid Weight Loss Plan

1. Enjoy 2 to 3 Revival milk protein or soy protein bars and shakes.
**EQUALS 400 – 600 calories.**
2. Enjoy 5 servings of fruits and vegetables of your choice.
**EQUALS 400 calories.**
3. Enjoy 1 low-calorie meal or pre-packaged entrée of your choice.
**EQUALS 200 – 300 calories.**
**BONUS SNACKS**: Enjoy 2 Revival snacks substituted for 1 bar or shake.
**EQUALS 200 calories** (about 100 calories per snack)
**TOTAL CALORIE COUNT**: About 1200 calories

- Drink calorie-free liquids (e.g., water, tea and diet soda) or enjoy calorie-containing drinks (e.g., natural fruit juices) as substitutes for a fruit and vegetable serving.
- Take a good multivitamin rich in antioxidants and beautifying ingredients.
- Walk 30 to 45 minutes, six days a week (or other physical activity that you enjoy) to burn an extra 2500 calories or more per week.
- Feeling hungry on 1200 calories per day? Increase calorie intake to 1400 to 1600 per day by adding in additional food items. This will keep your weight loss going at a slower rate versus a complete halt in progress.
- Use one naturally concentrated Revival soy bar or shake for full beauty and health benefits.

## My Favorite Rapid Weight Loss Daily Eating Pattern

**BREAKFAST:** a Revival shake blended with frozen fruit

**MID-MORNING BREAK:** a piece of fruit (e.g., a crisp apple)

**LUNCH:** a chocolate Revival bar and Revival protein chips

**MID-AFTERNOON BREAK:** a salty Revival snack

**DINNER:** a hot entrée with two steaming vegetables

*Alternate:* Revival pasta with two steaming vegetables

**NIGHTTIME SNACK:** bowl of frozen fruit medley

**FLUIDS:** as much calorie-free fluids as desired

**TOTAL FOOD COUNT:** 2 bars/shakes, 5 fruits/veggies, 1 entrée and
2 snacks

NOTE: Any 100-calorie snack can be substituted for a Revival snack.

**TOTAL CALORIE COUNT:** About 1200 calories

Daily eating pattern templates for you to personalize your pattern are
included in the next resource section.

## Weight Maintenance Plan

1. Enjoy 1 to 2 Revival milk protein or soy protein bars and shakes.
**EQUALS 200 – 400 calories.**
2. Enjoy 5 servings of fruits and vegetables of your choice.
**EQUALS 400 calories.**
3. Enjoy 2 low-calorie meals or pre-packaged entrées OR 1 sensible
   meals.
**EQUALS 400 – 800 calories.**
**BONUS SNACKS**: Enjoy 2 to 4 Revival snacks (or any 100-calorie
   snack)
**EQUALS 200 – 400 calories.**
**TOTAL CALORIE COUNT**: About 1800 – 2000 calories

- Most people find their sweet spot for weight maintenance to be
  between 1,800 to 2,000 calories per day.
- If you gain weight on 1800 to 2000 calories per day, make a slight
  adjustment to reduce calories by cutting out a snack or decreasing
  the calorie content of an entrée. You can also increase your physical activity level to burn more calories.
- Use one naturally concentrated Revival soy bar or shake for full
  beauty and health benefits.

## My Favorite Weight Maintenance Daily Eating Pattern

**BREAKFAST:** a Revival shake blended with frozen fruit

**MID-MORNING BREAK:** a piece of fruit and Revival protein chips

**LUNCH:** a hot entrée with a steaming vegetable

**MID-AFTERNOON BREAK:** a chocolate Revival bar and salty snack

**DINNER:** a hot entrée with two steaming vegetables

*Alternate:* Revival pasta with two steaming vegetables

**NIGHTTIME SNACK:** a sweet Revival snack and salty snack

**FLUIDS:** as much calorie-free fluids as desired

**TOTAL FOOD COUNT:** 2 bars/shakes, 5 fruits/veggies, 2 entrées, and 4 snacks

NOTE: Any 100-calorie snack can be substituted for a Revival snack!

**TOTAL CALORIE COUNT:** About 1800 – 2000 calories

## C. DAILY EATING PATTERN TEMPLATES

Personalizing your daily eating pattern for rapid weight loss or weight maintenance is easy with the templates below. Write it down and add it up. I recommend making extra blank photocopies before starting, or download blank templates at **www.RevivalDiet.com/Resources**.

Please contact my nutrition staff if you need help! And remember that my online diet management program (also at www.RevivalDiet.com) will help maximize your results.

---

**Rapid Weight Loss Daily Eating Pattern**

**Your TOTAL FOOD COUNT should be equivalent to the following:**

- 2 to 3 Revival milk protein or soy protein bars and shakes
- 5 servings of fruits and vegetables of your choice
- 1 low-calorie meal or pre-packaged entrée of your choice
- BONUS SNACKS: 2 Revival snacks substituted for 1 bar or shake

**BREAKFAST:**
**MID-MORNING BREAK:**
**LUNCH:**
**MID-AFTERNOON BREAK:**
**DINNER:**
**NIGHTTIME SNACK:**
**FLUIDS:**
**TOTAL FOOD COUNT:**
NOTE: Any 100-calorie snack can be substituted for a Revival snack.
**TOTAL CALORIE COUNT:** About 1200 calories

---

## Weight Maintenance Daily Eating Pattern

**Your TOTAL FOOD COUNT should be equivalent to the following:**

- 1 to 2 Revival milk protein or soy protein bars and shakes
- 5 servings of fruits and vegetables of your choice
- 2 low-calorie meals or pre-packaged entrées OR 1 sensible meal
- BONUS SNACKS: 2 to 4 Revival snacks (or any 100-calorie snack)

**BREAKFAST:**

**MID-MORNING BREAK:**

**LUNCH:**

**MID-AFTERNOON BREAK:**

**DINNER:**

**NIGHTTIME SNACK:**

**FLUIDS:**

**TOTAL FOOD COUNT:**

NOTE: Any 100-calorie snack can be substituted for a Revival snack!

**TOTAL CALORIE COUNT:** About 1800 – 2000 calories

# D. MEDICAL STUDY REFERENCES
# FOR THE INTELLECTUALLY CURIOUS

**NOTE:** These statements have not been evaluated by the Food and Drug Administration. Revival is not intended to diagnose, treat, cure, or prevent any disease. Study titles are not meant to imply treatment, curative, or preventative benefits.

### Weight Loss and Low-Glycemic Health Support

Anderson, J.W., J. Fuller, K. Patterson, R. Blair, and A. Tabor. Soy compared to casein meal replacement shakes with energy-restricted diets for obese women: randomized, controlled trial. Metabolism 2007; 56:280-288.

Blair RM, Tabor A, Henley EC. Soy foods have low glycemic and insulin response indices in normal weight subjects. Nutrition Journal 2006; 5:35.

Sites CK, Cooper BC, Gastaldelli A, Arabshahi A, Ridzon S, Cliver SP. Effect of daily supplement of soy phytoestrogens on body composition and insulin secretion in post-menopausal women. 2006 Annual Meeting of the American Society for Reproductive Medicine, October 21-25, 2006, New Orleans, LA.

Sydney University's Glycaemic Index Research Service. The glycaemic and insulin index values of six soy-based foods. A Glycaemic Index Research Report for Physicians Pharmaceuticals, July 2004.

Allison DB, Gadbury G, Schwartz LG, Murugesan R, Kraker JL, Heshka S, Fontaine KR, Heymsfield SB. A novel soy-based meal replacement formula for weight loss among obese individuals: a randomized controlled clinical trial. European Journal of Clinical Nutrition 2003; 57:514-522.

Anderson JW, Luan J, Hoie LH. Structured weight-loss programs: meta-analysis of weight loss at 24 weeks and assessment of effects of intervention intensity. Adv Ther. 2004; 21:61-75

Deibert P, Konig D, Schmidt-Trucksaess A, Zaenker KS, Frey I, Landmann U, Berg A. Weight loss without losing muscle mass in pre-obese and obese subjects induced by a high-soy-protein diet. International Journal of Obesity 2004; 28:1349-1352.

Eisenstein J, Roberts SB, Dallal G, Saltzman E. High-protein weight-loss diets: are they safe and do they work? A review of the experimental and epidemiologic data. Nutr Rev 2002; 60:189-200

Fontaine KR, Yang D, Gadbury GL, Heshka S, Schwartz LG, Murugesan R, Kraker JL, Heo M, Heymsfield SB, Allison DB. Results of a soy-based meal replacement formula on weight, anthropometry, serum lipids & blood pressure during a 40-week clinical weight loss trial. BMC Nutrition Journal 2003; 2:14-20.

Ludwig DS. The glycemic index: physiological mechanisms relating to obesity, diabetes and cardiovascular disease. JAMA 2002; 287:2414-2423.

Nishi T, Hara H, Tomita F. Soybean ,-conglycinin peptone suppresses food intake and gastric emptying by increasing plasma cholecystokinin levels in rats. Journal of Nutrition 2003; 133:352-357

### Energy & Exercise Health Support

Barbul A. The use of arginine in clinical practice. In: Cynober, LA, ed. Amino acid metabolism and therapy in health and nutritional disease. New York, NY. CRC Press Inc. 1998; pp. 361-383.

Box W, Hill S, DiSilvestro RA. Soy intake plus moderate weight resistance exercise: effects on serum concentrations of lipid peroxides in young adult women. Journal of Sports Medicine and Physical Fitness 2005; 45:524-528.

Brown EC, DiSilvestro RA, Babaknia A, Devor ST. Soy versus whey protein bars: effects on exercise training impact on lean body mass and antioxidant status. Nutrition Journal 2004; 3:22-26.

Chen CY, Bakhiet RM, Hart V, Holtzman G. Isoflavones improve plasma homocysteine status and antioxidant defense system in healthy young men at rest but do not ameliorate oxidative stress inducedc by 80% VO2pk exercise. Annals of Nutrition & Metabolism 2005; 49:33-41.

Djuric Z, Chen G, Doerge DR, Heilbrun LK, Kucuk O. Effect of soy isoflavone supplementation on markers of oxidative stress in men and women. Cancer Lett 2001; 172:1-6.

Hill S, Box W, DiSilvestro RA. Moderate intensity resistance exercise, plus or minus soy intake: effects on serum lipid peroxides in young adult males. International Journal of Sport Nutrition and Exercise Metabolism 2004; 14:125-132.

Parry-Billings M, Blomstrand E, McAndrew N, Newsholme EA. A communicational link between skeletal muscle, brain, and cells of the immune system. Int J Sports Med 1990; 2:S122-S128.

Rossi A, DiSilvestro RA, Blostein-Fujii. Effects of soy consumption on exercise induced acute muscle damage and oxidative stress in young adult males. FASEB 1998; 12(5):A653.

### Menopause Discomforts Health Support

Appling S, Kelly K, Allen J. Impact of Soy on Menopausal Symptoms. 17th Annual Conference of the Southern Nursing Research Society (SNRS), Orlando, Florida, February 2003.

Dupree K, Basaria S, Ojumu A, Bruno TW, John M, Wisniewski A, Dobs AS. Effects of soy on quality of life in post-menopausal women. The Endocrine Society Annual Meeting 2005, San Diego, CA, June 4 – 7.

Albertazzi P, Pansini F, Bonaccorsi G, Zanotti L, Forini E, de Aloysio D. The effect of dietary soy supplementation on hot flushes. Obstetrics & Gynecology 1998; 91:6-11.

Albertazzi P, Steel SA, Bottazzi M. Effect of pure genistein on bone markers and hot flushes. Climacteric 2005; 8:371-379.

Faure ED, Chantre P, Mares P. Effects of a standardized soy extract on hot flushes: a multicenter, double-blind, randomized, placebo-controlled study. Menopause 2002; 9:329-334.

Han KK, Soares Jr. JM, Haidar MA, Rodrigues de Lima G, Baracat EC. Benefits of soy isoflavone therapeutic regimen on menopausal symptoms. Obstetrics & Gynecology 2002; 99:389-394.

Jou HJ, Ling PY, Wu SC. Comparison of 70 mg and 35 mg isoflavone soya supplement for menopause symptoms. International Journal of Gynecology & Obstetrics 2005; 90:159-160.

Kaari C, Haidar MA, Soares Jr. JM, Nunes MG, de Azevedo Quadros LG, Kemp C, Stavale JN, Baracat EC. Randomized clinical trial comparing conjugated equine estrogens and isoflavones in postmenopausal women: a pilot study. Maturitas 2006; 53:49-58.

Kurzer M, Morgan T, Greaves K. Soy Isoflavones Decrease Hot-Flash Frequency: A Meta-Analysis of Studies Examining Soy Protein, Soyfood, and Soy Isoflavones. 5th International Symposium on the Role of Soy in Preventing and Treating Chronic Disease, Sept. 21-24th, 2003. Orlando, FL.

Morelli V, Naquin C. Alternative Therapies for Traditional Disease States: Menopause. American Family Physician 2002; 66:129-134.

Nagata C, Shimizu H, Takami R, Hayashi M, Takeda N, Yasuda K, Serum concentrations of estradiol and dehydroepiandrosterone sulfate and soy product intake in relation to psychologic well-being in peri- and postmenopausal Japanese women. Metabolism 2000; 49:1561-1564.

Nagata C, Takatsuka N, Kawakami N, Shimizu H. Soy product intake and hot flashes in Japanese women: Results from a community-based prospective study. Am J Epidemiol 2001; 153:790-793.

Ricciotti HA, Khaodhiar L, Blackburn GL. Daidzein-rich isoflavone-aglycones for menopausal symptoms. International Journal of Gynecology & Obstetrics 2005; 89:65-66.

Scambia G, Mango D, Signorile PG, Anselmi ARA, Palena C, Gallo D, Bombardelli E, Morazzoni P, Reva A, Mancuso S. Clinical effects of a standardized soy extract in postmenopausal women: a pilot study. Menopause 2000; 7:105-111.

Somekawa Y, Chiguchi M, Ishibashi T, Aso T. Soy intake related to menopausal symptoms, serum lipids, and bone mineral density in postmenopausal Japanese women. Obstetrics & Gynecology 2001; 97:109-115.

## Promotion of Normal PMS & Menstrual Health Support

Bryant M, Cassidy A, Hill C, Powell J, Talbot D, Dye L. Effect of consumption of soy isoflavones on behavioural, somatic and affective symptoms in women with premenstrual syndrome. British Journal of Nutrition 2005; 93:731-739.

Cassidy A, Bingham S, Setchell KD. Biological effects of a diet of soy protein rich in isoflavones on the menstrual cycle of premenopausal women. Am J Clin Nutr. 1994; 60:333-340.

Ishiwata N, Uesugi S, Uehara M, Watanabe S. Effects of Soy Isoflavones on Premenstrual Syndrome. 5th International Symposium on the Role of Soy in Preventing and Treating Chronic Disease, Sept. 21-24th, 2003. Orlando, FL.

Kumar NB, Cantor A, Allen K, Riccardi D, Cox CE. The specific role of isoflavones on estrogen metabolism in premenopausal women. Cancer 2002; 94:1166-1174.

Lu LJW, Anderson KE, Grady JJ, Kohen F, Nagamani M. Decreased ovarian hormones during a soya diet: implications for breast cancer prevention. Cancer Res 2000; 60:4112-4121.

Nagata C, Kabuto M, Kurisu Y, Shimizu H. Decreased serum estradiol concentration associated with high dietary intake of soy products in premenopausal Japanese women. Nutr Cancer 1997; 29:228-233.

Xu X, Duncan AM, Merz BE, Kurzer MS. Effects of soy isoflavones on estrogen and phytoestrogen metabolism in premenopausal women. Cancer Epidemiology Biomarkers Prev 1998; 7:1101-1108.

## Beautiful Skin, Hair & Nails Appearance Support

Draelos Z. The Effect of Revival Soy on the Health and Appearance of the Skin, Hair, and Nails in Postmenopausal Women. November 2005; Manuscript in Preparation.

DiSilvestro R. A Diversity of Soy Antioxidant Effects. 5th International Symposium on the Role of Soy in Preventing and Treating Chronic Disease, Sept. 21-24th, 2003. Orlando, FL.

Djuric Z, Chen G, Doerge DR, Heilbrun LK, Kucuk O. Effect of soy isoflavone supplementation on markers of oxidative stress in men and women. Cancer Lett 2001; 172:1-6

Kim SY, Kim SJ, Lee JY, Kim WG, Park WS, Sim YC, Lee SJ. Protective Effects of Dietary Soy Isoflavones against UV-Induced Skin-Aging in Hairless Mouse Model. J Am Coll Nutr 2004; 23:157-162.

Miyazaki K, Hanamizu T, Iizuka R, Chiba K. Genistein and daidzein stimulate hyaluronic acid production in transformed human keratinocyte culture and hairless mouse skin. Skin Pharmacol Appl Skin Physiol 2002; 15:175-183.

Moore JO, Wang Y, Stebbins WG, Gao D, Zhou X, Phelps R, Lebwohl M, Wei H. Photoprotective effect of isoflavone genistein on ultraviolet B induced pyrimidine dimmer formation and PCNA expression in human reconstituted skin and its implications in dermatology and prevention of cutaneous carcinogenesis. Carcinogenesis 2006: (Advance Access published March 7, 2006).

Reeve VE, WidyariniS, Domanski D, Chew E, Barnes K. Protection against photoaging in the hairless mouse by the isoflavone equol. Photochemistry and photobiology 2005; 81:1548-1553.

Skovgaard GRL, Jensen AS, Sigler ML. Effect of a novel dietary supplement on skin aging in post-menopausal women. European Journal of Clinical Nutrition 2006; (Advance online publication, May 3, 2006).

Sudel KM, Venzke K, Mielke H, Breitenbach U, Mundt C, Jaspers S, Koop U, Sauermann K, Knubmann-Hartig E, Moll I, Gercken G, Young AR, Stab F, Wenck H, Gallinat S. Novel aspects of intrinsic and extrinsic aging of human skin: beneficial effects of soy extract. Photochemistry and Photobiology 2005; 81:581-587.

Wei H, Saladi R, Lu Y, Wang Y, Palep SR, Moore J, Phelps R, Shyong E, Lebwohl MG. Isoflavone gensitein: photoprotection and clinical implications in dermatology. Journal of Nutrition 2003; 133:3811S-3819S.

Wei H, Zhang X, Wang Y, Lebwohl M. Inhibition of ultraviolet light-induced oxidative events in the skin and internal organs of hairless mice by isoflavone genistein. Cancer Letters 2002; 185:21-29.

Widyarini S, Allanson M, Gallagher NL, Pedley J, Boyle GM, Parsons PG, Whiteman DC, Walker C, Reeve VE. Isoflavonoid photoprotection in mouse and human skin is dependent on metallothionein. Journal of Investigative Dermatology 2006; 126:198-204.

## Promotion of Normal Cholesterol & Heart Health Support

Allen JK, Becker DM, Kwiterovich PO, Lindenstruth KA, Curtis C. Effect of soy protein-containing isoflavones on lipoproteins in postmenopausal women. Menopause 2006; 14: (In Press)

Allen, J.K. Soy and Lipoproteins in Postmenopausal Women. American Heart Association Scientific Sessions, November 2001, Anaheim, CA.

Anderson JW, Johnstone, BM, Cook-Newell ME. Meta-analysis of the effects of soy protein intake on serum lipids. New England Journal of Medicine 1995; 333:276-282.

Baum JA, Teng H, Erdman Jr JW, Weigel RM, Klein BP, Persky VW, Freels S, Surya P, Bakhit RM, Ramos E, Shay NF, Potter SM. Long-term intake of soy protein improves blood lipid profiles and increases mononuclear cell low-density-lipoprotein receptor messenger RNA in hypercholesterolemic, postmenopausal women. Am J Clin Nutr 1998; 68:545–551.

Bazzoli DL, Hill S, DiSilvestro RA. Soy protein antioxidant actions in active, young adult women. Nutrition Research 2002; 22:807-815.

Chacko BK, Chandler RT, Mundhekar A, Khoo N, Pruitt HM, Kucik DF, Parks DA, Kevil CG, Barnes S, Patel RP. Revealing anti-inflammatory mechanisms of soy isoflavones by flow: modulation of leukocyte-endothelial cell interactions. Am J Physiol Heart Circ Physiol 2005; 289:H908-H915.

Food and Drug Administration, U.S. Department of Health and Human Services, 1999. FDA TALK PAPER: FDA APPROVES NEW HEALTH CLAIM FOR SOY PROTEIN AND CORONARY HEART DISEASE: T99-48, October 20, 1999.

Hall WL, Vafeiadou K, Hallund J, Bugel S, Koebnick C, Reimann M, Ferrari M, Branca F, Talbot D, Dadd T, Nilsson M, Dahlman-Wright K, Gustafsson JA, Minihane AM, Williams CM. Soy-isoflavone-enriched foods and inflammatory biomarkers of cardiovascular disease risk in postmenopausal women: interactions with genotype and equol production. American Journal of Clinical Nutrition 2005; 82:1260-1268.

Hallund J, Bugel S, Tholstrup T, Ferrari M, Talbot D, Hall WL, Reimann M, Williams CM, Wiinberg N. Soy isoflavone-enriched cereal bars affect markers of endothelial function in postmenopausal women. British Journal of Nutrition 2006; 95:1120-1126.

Hodgson JM, Croft KD, Puddey IB, Mori TA, Beilin LJ. Soybean isoflavonoids and their metabolic products inhibit in vitro lipoprotein oxidation in serum. Journal of Nutritional Biochemistry 1996; 7:664-669.

Hwang J, Sevanian A, Hodis HN, Ursini F. Synergistic inhibition of LDL oxidation by phytoestrogens and ascorbic acid. Free Radical Biology & Medicine 2000; 29:79-89.

Jenkins DJ, Kendall CW, Jackson CJ, Connelly PW, Parker T, Faulkner D, Vidgen E, Cunnane SC, Leiter LA, Josse RG. Effects of high- and low-isoflavone soyfoods on blood lipids, oxidized LDL, homocysteine, and blood pressure in hyperlipidemic men and women. Am J Clin Nutr 2002; 76:365-372.

Merz CNB, Johnson BD, Braunstein GD, Pepine CJ, Reis SE, Paul-Labrador M, Hale G, Sharaf BL, Bittner V, Sopko G, Kelsey SF for the Women's Ischemia Syndrome Evaluation Study Group. Phytoestrogens and lipoproteins in women. Journal of Clinical Endocrinology & Metabolism 2006; 91:2209-2213.

Washburn S, Burke GL, Morgan T, Anthony M. Effect of soy protein supplementation

on serum lipoproteins, blood pressure, and menopausal symptoms in perimenopausal women. Menopause 1999; 6:7-13.

Wiseman H, O'Reilly JDO, Adlercreutz H, Mallet AI, Bowey EA, Rowland IR, Sanders
TAB. Isoflavone phytoestrogens consumed in soy decrease F2-isoprostane concentra-
tions and increase resistance of low-density lipoprotein to oxidation in humans.
American Journal of Clinical Nutrition 2000; 72:395-400.

Zhan S, Ho SC. Meta-analysis of the effects of soy protein containing isoflavones on the
lipid profile. American Journal of Clinical Nutrition 2005; 81:397-408.

Zhuo X-G, Melby MK, Watanabe S. Soy isoflavone intake lowers serum LDL cholesterol:
a meta-analysis of 8 randomized controlled trials in humans. Journal of Nutrition
2004; 134:2395-2400.

## Antioxidant Health Support

Aoki H, Otaka Y, Igarashi K, Takenaka A. Soy protein reduces paraquat-induced oxidative stress in rats. Journal of Nutrition 2002; 132:2258-2262.

Bazzoli DL, Hill S, DiSilvestro RA. Soy protein antioxidant actions in active, young adult
women. Nutrition Research 2002; 22:807-815.

Chen CY, Bakhiet RM, Hart V, Holtzman G. Isoflavones improve plasma homocysteine
status and antioxidant defense system in healthy young men at rest but do not ameliorate oxidative stress induced by 80% VO2pk exercise. Annals of Nutrition &
Metabolism 2005; 49:33-41.

Damasceno NRT, Goto H, Rodrigues FMD, Dia CTS, Okawabata FS, Abdalla DSP,
Gidlund M. Soy protein isolate reduces the oxidizability of LDL and the generation
of oxidized LDL autoantibodies in rabbits with diet-induced atherosclerosis. Journal
of Nutrition 2000; 130:2641-2647.

DiSilvestro R. A Diversity of Soy Antioxidant Effects. 5th International Symposium on
the Role of Soy in Preventing and Treating Chronic Disease, Sept. 21-24th, 2003,
Orlando, FL.

DiSilvestro RA, Goodman J, Dy E, LaValle G. Soy isoflavone supplementation elevates
erythrocyte superoxide dismutase, but not ceruloplasmin in postmenopausal breast
cancer survivors. Breast Cancer Research and Treatment 2005; 89:251-255.

Djuric Z, Chen G, Doerge DR, Heilbrun LK, Kucuk O. Effect of soy isoflavone supplementation on markers of oxidative stress in men and women. Cancer Letters 2001;
172:1-6.

Guo Q, Rimbach G, Moini H, Weber S, Packer L. ESR and cell culture studies on free
radical-scavenging and antioxidant activities of isoflavonoids. Toxicology 2002;
179:171-180.

Hodgson JM, Croft KD, Puddey IB, Mori TA, Beilin LJ. Soybean isoflavonoids and their
metabolic products inhibit in vitro lipoprotein oxidation in serum. Journal of
Nutritional Biochemistry 1996; 7:664-669.

Hwang J, Sevanian A, Hodis HN, Ursini F. Synergistic inhibition of LDL oxidation by
phytoestrogens and ascorbic acid. Free Radical Biology & Medicine 2000; 29:79-89.

Rimbach G, De Pascual-Teresa S, Weins BA, Matsugo S, Uchida Y, Minihane AM,
Turner R, Vafeiadou K, Weinberg, PD. Antioxidant and free radical scavenging
activity of isoflavone metabolites. Xenobiotica 2003; 33:913-925.

Wiseman H, O'Reilly JDO, Adlercreutz H, Mallet AI, Bowey EA, Rowland IR, Sanders TAB. Isoflavone phytoestrogens consumed in soy decrease F2-isoprostane concentrations and increase resistance of low-density lipoprotein to oxidation in humans. American Journal of Clinical Nutrition 2000; 72:395-400.

## Promotion of Normal Bone Health Support

Arjmandi BH, Khalil DA, Smith BJ, Lucas EA, Juma S, Payton ME, Wild RA. Soy protein has a greater effect on bone in postmenopausal women not on hormone replacement therapy, as evidenced by reducing bone resorption and urinary calcium excretion. J Clin Endocrinol Metab 2003; 88:1048-1054.

Arjmandi BH, Lucas EA, Khalil DA, Devareddy L, Smith BJ, McDonald J, Arquitt AB, Payton ME, Mason C. One year soy protein supplementation has positive effects on bone formation markers but not bone density in postmenopausal women. Nutrition Journal 2005; 4:8

Chiechi LM, Secreto G, D'Amore M, Fanelli M, Venturelli E, Cantatore F, Valerio T, Laselva G, Loizzi P. Efficacy of a soy rich diet in preventing postmenopausal osteoporosis: the Menfis randomized trial. Maturitas 2002; 42:295-300.

Ho SC, Guldan GS, Woo J, Yu R, Tse MM, Sham A, Cheng J. A prospective study of the effects of 1-year calcium-fortified soy milk supplementation on dietary calcium intake and bone health in Chinese adolescent girls aged 14-16. Osteoporosis International 2005; Advance Online Publication doi: 10.1007/s00198-005-1963-8

Horiuchi T, Onouchi T, Takahashi M, Ito H, Orimo H. Effect of soy protein on bone metabolism in postmenopausal Japanese women. Osteoporos Int 2000; 11:721-724.

Ikeda Y, Iki M, Morita A, Kajita E, Kagamimori S, Kagawa Y, Yoneshima H. Intake of fermented soybeans, Natto, is associated with reduced bone loss in postmenopausal women: Japanese Population-based Osteoporosis (JPOS) Study. J Nutr 2006; 136:1323-1328.

Messina M, Ho S, Alekel DL. Skeletal benefits of soy isoflavones: a review of the clinical trial and epidemiologic data. Curr Opin Clin Nutr Metab Care 2004; 7:649-658.

Morabito N, Crisafulli A, Vergara C, Gaudio A, Lasco A, Frisina N, D'Anna R, Corrado F, Pizzoleo MA, Cincotta M, Altavilla D, Ientile R, Squadrito F. Effects of genistein and hormone-replacement therapy on bone loss in early postmenopausal women: a randomized double-blind placebo-controlled study. Bone Miner Res 2002; 17:1904-1912.

Newton KM, LaCroix AZ, Levy L, Li SS, Qu P, Potter JD, Lampe JW. Soy protein and bone mineral density in older men and women: a randomized trial. Maturitas 2006; 55: 270-277.

Roudsari AH, Tahbaz F, Hossein-Nezhad A, Arjmandi B, Larijani B, Kimiagar SM. Assessment of soy phytoestrogens' effects on bone turnover indicators in menopausal women with osteopenia in Iran: a before and after clinical trial. Nutrition Journal 2005; 4:30

Scheiber MD, Liu JH, Subbiah MT, Rebar RW, Setchell KD. Dietary inclusion of whole soy foods results in significant reductions in clinical risk factors for osteoporosis and cardiovascular disease in normal postmenopausal women. Menopause 2001; 8:384-392.

Setchell KD, Lydeking-Olsen E. Dietary phytoestrogens and their effect on bone: evidence from in vitro and in vivo, human observational, and dietary intervention studies. Am J Clin Nutr 2003; 78(3 Suppl):593S-609S.

Somekawa Y, Chiguchi M, Ishibashi T, Aso T. Soy intake related to menopausal symptoms, serum lipids, and bone mineral density in postmenopausal Japanese women. Obstet Gynecol 2001; 97:109-115.

Ye YB, Tang XY, Verbruggen MA, Su YX. Soy isoflavones attenuate bone loss in early postmenopausal Chinese women. A single-blind randomized, placebo-controlled study. European Journal of Nutrition 2006; EPub ahead of print.

Zhang X, Shu XO, Li H, Yang G, Li Q, Gao YT, Zheng W. Prospective cohort study of soy food consumption and risk of bone fracture among postmenopausal women. Archives of Internal Medicine 2005; 165:1890-1895.

## Promotion of Normal Blood Sugar Health Support

Anderson JW, Blake JE, Turner J, Smith BM. Effects of soy protein on renal function and proteinuria in patients with type 2 diabetes. American Journal of Clinical Nutrition 1998; 68(6 Suppl):1347S-1353S.

Azadbakht L, Shakerhosseini R, Atabak S, Jamshidian M, mehrabi Y, Esmaill-Zadeh A. Beneficiary effect of dietary soy protein on lowering plasma levels of lipid and improving kidney function in type II diabetes with nephropathy. Eur J Clin Nutr 2003; 57:1292-1294.

Bhathena SJ, Velasquez MT. Beneficial role of dietary phytoestrogens in obesity and diabetes. Am J Clin Nutr 2002; 76:1191-1201.

Exner M, Hermann M, Hofbauer R, Kapiotis S, Quehenberger P, Speiser W, Held I, Gmeiner BM. Genistein prevents the glucose autoxidation mediated atherogenic modification of low density lipoprotein. Free Radic Res 2001; 34:101-112.

Jayagopal V, Albertazzi P, Kilpatrick ES, Howarth EM, Jennings PE, Hepburn DA, Atkin SL. Beneficial effects of soy phytoestrogen intake in postmenopausal women with type 2 diabetes. Diabetes Care 2002; 25:1709-1714.

Li Z, Hong K, Saltsman P, DeShields S, Bellman M, Thames G, Liu Y, Wang HJ, Elashoff R, Heber D. Long-term efficacy of soy-based meal replacements vs an individualized diet plan in obese type II DM patients: relative effects on weight loss, metabolic parameters, and C-reactive protein. European Journal of Clinical Nutrition 2005; 59:411-418.

## Promotion of Normal Memory Health Support

Casini ML, Marelli G, Papaleo E, Ferrrari A, D'Ambrosio F, Unfer V. Psychological assessment of the effects of treatment with phytoestrogens on postmenopausal women: a randomized, double-blind, crossover, placebo-controlled study. Fertility & Sterility 2006; 85:972-978.

Celec P, Ostatnikova D, Caganova M, Zuchova S, Hodosy J, Putz Z, Bernadic M, Kudela M. Endocrine and cognitive effects of short-time soybean consumption in women. Gynecologic and Obstetric Investigation 2005; 59:62-66.

Duffy R, Wiseman H, File SE. Improved cognitive function in postmenopausal women after 12 weeks of consumption of a soya extract containing isoflavones. Pharmacol Biochem Behav 2003; 75:721-729.

File SE, Hartley DE, Elsabagh S, Duffy R, Wiseman H. Cognitive improvement after 6 weeks of soy supplements in postmenopausal women is limited to frontal lobe function. Menopause 2005; 12:193-201.

File SE, Jarrett N, Fluck E, Duffy R, Casey K, Wiseman H. Eating soya improves human memory. Psychopharmacology (Berl) 2001; 157:430-436.

Heo HJ, Suh YM, Kim MJ, Choi SJ, Mun NS, Kim HK, Kim E, Kim CJ, Cho HY, Kim YJ, Shin DH. Daidzein activates choline acetyltransferase from MC-IXC cells and improves drug-induced amnesia. Biosci Biotechnol Biochem 2006; 70:107-111.

Kim H, et al. Modulation of Neurodegeneration Markers by Dietary Soy in a Primate Model of Menopause. 3rd International Symposium on the Role of Soy in Preventing and Treating Chronic Disease, Oct. 31 – Nov. 3, 1999, Washington, DC.

Kim H, Xia H, Li L, Gewin J. Attenuation of neurodegeneration-relevant modifications of brain proteins by dietary soy. Biofactors 2000; 12:243-250.

Kritz-Silverstein D, von Muhlen D, Barrett-Connor E, Bressel MAB. Isoflavones and cognitive function in older women: the Soy and Postmenopausal Health In Aging (SOPHIA) study. Menopause 2003; 10:196-202.

## Milk Protein Benefits for Weight Loss and Promotion of Normal Bone Health Support

Boon N, Hul GBJ, Viguerie N, Sicard A, Langin D, Saris WHM. Effects of 3 diets with various calcium contents on 24-h energy expenditure, fat oxidation, and adipose tissue message RNA expression of lipid metabolism-related proteins. American Journal of Clinical Nutrition. 2005; 82: 1244-52.

Chan She Ping-Delfos W, Soares MJ, Cummings NK. Acute suppression of spontaneous food intake following dairy calcium and vitamin D. Nutrition Society of Australia Annual Conference. Asia Pacific Journal of Clinical Nutrition. 2004;13. Abstract.

Davies KM, et al. Calcium intake and body weight. Journal of Clinical Endocrinology & Metabolism. 2000; 85(12): 4635-4638.

Gunther CW, Legowski PA, Lyle RM, McCabe GP, Eagan MS, Peacock M, Teegarden D. Dairy products do not lead to alterations in body weight and fat mass in young women in a one year intervention. American Journal of Clinical Nutrition. 2005; 81(4): 751-6.

Gunther CW, Lyle RM, Legowski PA, James JM, McCabe LD, McCabe GP, Peacock M, Teegarden D. Fat oxidation and its relation to serum parathyroid hormone in young women enrolled in a 1-y dairy calcium intervention. American Journal of Clinical Nutrition. 2005; 82: 1228-1234.

Harvey-Berino J, et al. The impact of calcium and dairy product consumption on weight loss. Obesity Research. 2005; 13; 1720-1726.

Heaney RP, et al. Normalizing calcium intake: Projected population effects for body weight. Journal of Nutrition. 2003; 133:268S-270S.

Hirota T, Kawasaki I, Ikeda H, Aoe T, Hirota K. Intake of vitamin D and milk was associated with increase in muscle mass and decrease in body fat during dieting in young women. American Society for Bone and Mineral Research Annual Meeting. 2005. Abstract M272.

Jacobsen R, et al. Effect of short-term high dietary calcium intake on 24-h energy expenditure, fat oxidation, and fecal fat excretion. International Journal of Obesity. 2005; 29: 292-301.

Kalkwarf HJ, et al. Milk intake during childhood and adolescence, adult bone density, and osteoporotic fractures in US women. American Journal of Clinical Nutrition. 2003; 77: 257-265.

Kim D, Rhee Y, Ahn C, Cha B, Kim K, Lee H, Lim S. Effects of calcium supplementation on body composition and fat distribution in Korean obese postmenopausal women. American Society for Bone and Mineral Research Annual Meeting. 2005. Abstract SA422.

Lin YC, et al. Dairy calcium is related to changes in body composition during a two-year exercise intervention in young women. Journal of the American College of Nutrition. 2000; 19(6):754-760.

Melanson EL, Donahoo WT, Dong F, Ida T, Zemel MB. Effect of low- and high-calcium dairy-based diets on macronutrient oxidation in humans. Obesity Research. 2005;13:2102-12.

Melton LJ, et al. Relative contributions of bone density, bone turnover, and clinical risk factors to long-term fracture prediction. Journal of Bone and Mineral Research. 2003; 18: 312-318.

Munger RG, et al. Prospective study of dietary protein intake and risk of hip fracture in postmenopausal women. American Journal of Clinical Nutrition. 1999; 69: 147-152.

Teegarden D, et al. Dietary calcium intake protects women consuming oral contraceptives from spine and hip bone loss. Journal of Clinical Endocrinology and Metabolism. 2005.

Thompson WG, Holdman NR, Janzow DJ, Slezak JM, Morris KL, Zemel MB. Effect of energy-reduced diets high in dairy products and fiber on weight loss in obese adults. Obesity Research. 2005; 13:1344-1353.

U.S Department of Health and Human Services. Bone Health and Osteoporosis: A Report of the Surgeon General. Rockville, MD: US Department of Health and Human Services, Office of the Surgeon General, 2004.

Zemel MB, Teegarden D, Van Loan M., Schoeller DA., Matkovic V., Lyle RM., Craig BA. Role of dairy products in modulating weight and fat loss: A multi-center trial. FASEB J. 2004; 18(5): A845. Abstract.

Zemel MB, Thompson W, Milstead A, Morris K, Campbell P. Calcium and dairy acceleration of weight and fat loss during energy restriction in obese adults. Obesity Research. 2004; 12(4): 582-590.

Zemel MB, Richards J, Russel J, Milstead A, Gehardt L, Silva E. Dairy augmentation of total and central fat loss in obese subjects. International Journal of Obesity. 2005; 29(4):341-7.

Zemel MB, Richards J, Milstead A, Campbell P. Effects of calcium and dairy on body composition and weight loss in African-American adults. Obesity Research. 2005 13(7): 1218-1225.

## E. HEALTHCARE PROVIDER PATIENT SAMPLES PROGRAM

You can join thousands of physicians, dietitians, and other healthcare providers that have already recommended Revival products to their patients. Our clinically proven natural solutions are a solid addition to any patient's overall healthcare plan.

Free patient samples and educational brochures are available by contacting us at 1-800-500-8053. Visit **www.RevivalDiet.com/Medical** for more information.

Alternately, if you don't want to hand out samples or brochures, you can simply refer patients to 1-800-REVIVAL or www.RevivalDiet.com.

If you would like to sell Revival products in your medical office, spa or pharmacy, please contact us. We appreciate your interest in Revival. Dr. Tabor and Revival's nutrition staff are available to answer your questions.

*Together we can change the world—one patient at a time!*

## F. NUTRITION STAFF AND ORDER INFORMATION

We are here to serve you with good nutrition, education, and medical research to help you live a life you love. It's super easy to start because my nutrition staff will help you select the perfect *Revival Slim & Beautiful Diet* package containing all of the exact products you need. Please contact us if you have questions!

**Nutrition Staff and Order Center**
**PHONE:** 1-800-REVIVAL (1-800-738-4825)
**WEBSITE & ONLINE DIET MANANGEMENT:** www.RevivalDiet.com
**FREE NEWSLETTER AND BLOG:** www.RevivalDiet.com/News
**EMAIL:** Nutrition@RevivalDiet.com

**Aaron Tabor, MD**
CEO and Medical Research Director
Physicians Laboratories
**E-MAIL:** Doc@RevivalDiet.com
**PHONE:** 1-800-REVIVAL (1-800-738-4825)
**FAX:** 336-722-7712

**Suzanne Tabor, "Dr. Mom"**
President and CFO
Physicians Laboratories
**E-MAIL:** Mom@RevivalDiet.com

We've prepared a special video welcome message for you.
Watch it today at **www.RevivalDiet.com**.